THE SECRET CURE TO BACK PAIN

How to Avoid a Life of Painkillers and Surgery

DR JEREMY ANDREWS
(DOCTOR OF CHIROPRACTIC)

TABLE OF CONTENTS

Introduction 1

The complicated spine 5

What causes back pain 11

Why do some people get pain and others don't 19

The number one mistake with back pain 25

Why does it always come back? 33

How to resolve back pain 45

The secret remedy to getting rid of back pain for good 85

What's the difference between Chiropractors, Osteopaths, and Physiotherapists? 89

'I'm too old to get my back fixed' 93

The most common questions my clients ask 97

What do our clients say? 101

Introduction

If you are reading this you probably have tried a number of different methods to fix your back pain and become pretty frustrated, and I'm guessing it hasn't been going on for just a few days; it may be months or years.

Thank you so much for picking up my book. I really appreciate you taking the time. This is packed full of useful tips and tricks to help with chronic long-term spinal pain.

I have a disclaimer, I wrote this book myself without the help of a ghost writer or publisher. So any slights of language or grammar, please accept this apology now. English never was a strong subject for me.

It may be that one of our clients has sent this to you and insisted that you read it. Firstly, I know it's hard to find time to often read books, but if you are suffering with back or neck pain, I have seen over 30,000 different cases. I haven't seen it all, but I have a good idea of what techniques work best and what doesn't. Everyone is different, and research and techniques are always evolving as we get better each year at treating back pain. So take an hour or two and ingest some life changing information. You may know some of the techniques already, but my pledge to you is that if you apply what you see in this book, you will be in a better position in a month's time than you are now.

Why did I decide to write a book about back pain? It was something that I have lived and breathed for the past ten years. I started seeing some patterns and thought I could be on to something. Then I had the stark realisation that there was no 'one-size' fits all approach to back pain. It requires individual attention and analysis, working closely with each client to get to the root cause of the issue and prevent long-term problems. I'm fascinated with the spine and its many interactions; I hope reading this book will shed some light on your spinal issues and guide you to better days ahead.

All of the cases I talk about in the book are clients that I have treated over the years, their names and ages have been changed.

So, I originally grew up in a small town in Surrey called Haslemere. I went to school in Petersfield where I played lots of sport, particularly hockey, cricket, football, and the occasional game of rugby. However, I must admit that even being at a rugby school I didn't get on with the physicality. Hockey was fast and skilful, somewhat slightly better suited to my appetite. Not saying I'm either of these, but better suited than rugby.

At school I developed a passion for Biology, and it was one of the few subjects I enjoyed and therefore did reasonably well at. I took it at A-level and had some great teachers and peers who advised me to take a degree in Human Musculoskeletal Science at the University of Bristol, which began in 2007.

Bristol was a great three years; lots going on, trendy, and a city on the up. I played a lot of hockey, had a few late nights and got stuck to my studies. The first year was mainly mammalian anatomy and physiology, a pharmacology module and one in physiology. My final year I specialised in bones and the spine. I did a dissertation where I looked at trying to disprove the gold standard of assessing the integrity of bone called DEXA.

This final year prepared me well for a career in Chiropractic . I finished my undergraduate in 2010 and started my Masters of Chiropractic that Autumn.

Bournemouth was the destination, and now a 'mature' student, the world was my oyster. A mature twenty-one year old had a blast: beach, the New Forest, and a few more late nights and much more studying over the next four years paved the way. Chiropractic college is a tough gig, and anyone who says otherwise is lying. The final year I spent in the clinic on site at the college where you have to deliver 400 treatments and the right learning procedures and reports for each of them before you can get your degree. Fortunately, everything went off without a hitch apart from a minor wrist fracture that left me unable to practice for four months, but that is neither here nor there.

I had a very fortunate educational career which has led me on a specific path to working with something that I'm incredibly passionate about, always learning new skills of how to treat different patients, and adapt to the ever growing research being produced regarding the spine.

I can now be found in my clinic in West Byfleet, Surrey with my three chiropractic associates, totalling a team of nine in the clinic.

Thank you to Charlotte; you are incredible, to Kit; you are so special, and to Mum and Dad for all your support.

The Complicated Spine

The spine is an incredibly complex structure. If you ask anyone that has worked with the spine for years, they will tell you that no one patient is the same. Somebody with a textbook problem on an MRI will present completely different to the next person and that is why spinal treatment comes with its challenges.

That being said, we are much further along than where we were thirty years ago. Knowledge was very limited as to how the spine functioned, and it's only after years of monitoring chronic pain patients with high disability and lack of independence that we now know more about how the biomechanics of the spine works.

Many of you reading this book will know someone, or you may be suffering yourselves, with chronic back pain. Low back pain continues to be one of the highest sources of disability worldwide. Almost every single adult in the developed world will experience back pain at some stage throughout their life to a varying degree.

Many spinal surgeons will try and defer spinal surgery for as long as possible. The reason being that many patients stay the same following a five-year follow-up review and many get worse.

This is because the spine is such an intricate structure, and when you change one portion it causes a dramatic effect on the rest of the spine. Many of you reading this will have had or know someone who has had spinal surgery and will have had differing results. Generally, one of the most common surgeries in the spine is a microdiscectomy. This tends to be in younger males and is where there is a disc injury in the lower portion of the spine. The surgeon will locate the disc where it has slipped—the scientific term is called herniation —he will then take this portion of the disc off. This can yield fantastic results immediately because the pressure has been taken off the nerve and the surrounding structures. It's not till months or even years afterwards that the biomechanics of the spine will be altered and could cause a knock-on effect elsewhere. It's not uncommon for people who have had one microdiscectomy to have a second purely because the other discs have to take up more weight.

The lower disc called the L5/S1 disc is the most common disc to herniate because it takes up the most weight. It is the biggest disc and therefore causes the most amount of problems. Discs will usually be herniated to the side and will press on the nerves going into the back and down the legs, often causing sciatica. Sciatica is where there is pressure from a disc which can cause shooting searing pain down the back of the leg all the way to the toes. This is not limited to a shooting pain; it can present itself as pins and needles, numbness, or lack of control or strength in the leg.

If this is the case with lots of preoperative patients, then a microdiscectomy taking pressure off the disc can immediately relieve stress on the sciatic nerve taking the pain away, allowing the patient to restore normal capability. The L4/5 disc is the one above and now will begin to take up more of the load bearing from the chest, the shoulders and the head.

Little does the patient know, that this disc will eventually degenerate as well. It could be a year, could be ten years, it could be thirty years, but it's not designed to take up the enormous amounts of stress the body will place upon it.

That being said every human judges how healthy they are by the way they feel, and this is how we automatically determine how our bodies are functioning. If there is no pain, we go back to doing the things we did before the operation. For example, a young rugby player who has a disc injury will avoid doing any gym work, weight-lifting, or running for fear of causing debilitating pain. He has surgery, and the pressure will come off the spine and sciatic nerve. It will allow him to return to normal activity, only placing more stress and force through an unstable spine.

Spinal surgeons will always try and delay any sort of surgery in the back for as long as possible and try to restore normal motion and pain free mobility through non-surgical methods.

Another very important structure in the spine is the spinal cord and the column which it runs through. The spinal cord is elastic, designed to bend, stretch and flex as the spine does when we go through our daily activities such as sitting, twisting, and walking up and downstairs. It sends motor neurons from the brain, signalling to our body commands such as to lift a pencil up or to lift that glass of water. Going the other way, we have sensory nerves providing information to the brain about temperature and pain.

If this structure becomes compressed or compromised, that is when we start to experience dysfunction, whether it be pain, pins and needles, numbness, hot and cold, or the inability to move as we desire. The spinal cord will exit at each level throughout the spinal column, and then branch with roots to the subsequent endpoints, like a river with its tributaries.

With the degeneration in the spine often the spinal column itself can become smaller with time and arthritic damage, and the exit points from the side of the vertebra can also become smaller. What this does is put pressure on the nerve, and when a nerve has pressure on it, it won't be able to function as it normally does, thus creating symptoms.

There are twenty-four vertebrae in the spinal column, seven in the neck, twelve in the thoracic region, and five in the lumbar region. At the base of the spine there is a fused bone called the sacrum, which leads into the coccyx, often referred to as the tailbone. Originally, many thousands of years ago, we did have tails but with evolution this has changed into a small fused coccyx at the base of the buttocks. The spine is designed to be curved from the side to give springy shock absorption when we are lifting, bending and twisting, and it's supposed to be straight when we look at a patient from the front.

With 21st century demands, the spine and its curves will change and cause different weight distributions to go through different areas and this is one of the main causes of arthritic bony change. The most common change in the spine we see is something called a forward head carriage where the cervical curve starts to straighten the head and starts to move forwards making the chin jut out . This is because of sitting for long periods, working behind computers and the emergence of the smartphone. The head is the weight of a bowling ball, if we start to lose the cervical curve it puts pressure on the front of the bones in the neck. This can then cause the cervical discs to come under stress including cervical disc herniations which are incredibly difficult to fix due to a close proximity to vital arteries and nerves running in the neck.

The spine moves in every direction and does what it is designed to do, which is provide support for the rest of the body. If we didn't have a spine, there would be nothing for muscles and ribs to attach to and no protection for vital organs including the heart, lungs, liver, and pancreas.

What Causes Back Pain

Traditionally, thousands of years ago, our ancestors were upright cavemen with huge back muscles and huge, big buttock muscles. As we have developed and evolved over time, we have been forced to spend long periods during the day behind desks with computers, and also driving. This is causing spinal problems to increase rapidly. To give an example, we now see children as young as twelve years old with signs of arthritic change.

Billions of pounds have been spent on spinal research attempting to answer the question why do people get back pain? Why do some people get back pain and sometimes have certain conditions? How it works over a long period of time? Our bodies are complex machines. We will never change, the way we work has just changed.

This is incredibly alarming for many reasons. We only have one spine, it's not like we can do a spine transplant. Do you start to mess around with the spine from a surgical point of view? If you ask any spinal surgeon they will always try and avoid the risk of surgery. Orthopaedic surgeons who specialise in spine surgery will say it is always the last resort. Leave the way the spine functions in each individual to each person.

We also need to remember that the back is the centre of a seesaw, as it were. What I mean by that, is that it is integral to the way that we move, walk, sit, and lie; there is no rest or let up for the back, and there are constant demands on it to be active. It links the legs and torso and head and keeps us upright.

So, although bad positioning or injuries can cause a back issue directly, it's also common to get an injury from an imbalance elsewhere in the body.

Diane is one of our clients who has been with us for over a year now. She is 55 and an avid marathon runner for the last ten years. She has had an ongoing hip and pelvic issue for the past five years, which is managed with stretching, massage, physiotherapy, and acupuncture.

She responds very well to these treatments. Although her pain is under control and she can still train for marathons without the pelvic pain causing disability, she came to me and asked why the pain kept recurring and what was causing the issue?

It gets me excited to meet those with a chronic issue who have already had treatment. It means that the other experts have done a fantastic job at managing the issue but haven't managed to locate the root cause of the problem which is why it never resolves. I can't emphasise enough the importance of analysing the whole body from a holistic point of view to identify exactly why the problem is carrying on. Some people get frustrated with us as we have such a vigorous two-day process before we make any adjustments or treatment to ensure that we have all the information so we can provide the best treatment. We often hear "Can't you just treat me now?" to which I respond "Yes of course we can, but we haven't got the information yet and it's purely guesswork, you wouldn't want a heart surgeon to guess with your heart health or a brain surgeon to guess with your brain health so let's take the next 24 hours to prepare a plan with specific goals along the way and expectations we need to hit with the full diagnostics."

So when Diane presented I automatically needed to look elsewhere in the body; she was always getting care for her pelvis and hip issue. The cause of a lot of pelvic and hip issues can often be instability through the base of the spine, and especially in women who have children this is common due to the amount of stress that pregnancy will put through the body. In this case, because Diane was running twenty miles a week for the last ten years, a good place to start would be the leg and the foot.

We analysed range of motion throughout the knee joint, ankle joint, and the foot bones. The reason being that the foot on the ankle has many tiny bones that will grip and move as someone goes through a gait cycle, let alone twenty miles a week. On the ankle there is a bone that sits underneath the lower leg and ankle; it is a platform for the foot to spring off and with Diane it was not moving properly. This causes the right leg to work a lot harder when moving and running, tightening up the muscles around the upper leg and buttocks, pulling the pelvis across, causing an opposite strain around the left hip and buttock area. The body is amazing at compensating for problems and often you will see this pattern where the root issue is on one side and the pain is on the other.

So, we adjusted the foot to free up the bone and worked on getting the pelvis stable as well. If we just stabilised the pelvis with adjustments and core stability exercises, the problem would have kept coming back when she went back to running. With the ankle freed up, it could go through the full gait range and go through the normal cycle, thus creating pain free running and more marathons for Diane to complete.

It's really important to remember that we have to look at the whole body when analysing any sort of problem. All too often as experts we can get honed-in on the pain and lose sight of the bigger picture. We often see clients that have had chronic pain for ten-twenty years and seen multiple experts; this is where we usually see these problems.

This next one is often more difficult for people to understand. When we go through our new patient process, they will ask a series of questions to direct the examination procedure. One of the questions is "Can you think of anything that's happened in the past that could be playing a role into why you got this pain?" The most common response is "No, it just started."

As human beings, we are conditioned to block out painful episodes, otherwise we would never try new things. It's only when we delve deeper and ask more specific questions about falls, accidents, injuries, and car crashes that we begin to get more of an idea of what caused the back pain.

We have a lovely client called Emma in the clinic who is 41 and a carer. She was referred in by her father and sister who also come to the clinic. She presented with cluster headaches. This is a recurrent headache and often they can come up to thirty times in an hour and be persistent throughout the day. They are incredibly debilitating and can destroy people's daily life.

We began the medical history with Emma and asked her what she thought could be causing them, she couldn't think why, as they just came on one night. I began asking her questions about injuries and accidents, and when I asked her about any car accidents she remembered one that she had fifteen years ago in her 20s. She was at a traffic light and someone skidded and came into the back of her and hit her at 40 mph. There was significant damage to the car but fortunately no one was hurt.

I asked Emma what position her head was in at the time of the accident — usually our clients do not remember. But Emma remembered vividly; she was looking out of the window at a couple of kids at the lights who were messing around. This is vital because when you have any sort of accident if there is twisting or rotation in the spine it can make the issue a lot worse. She had her head turned to the side with a whiplash injury which will cause long term ligament damage and changes in the structure of the neck. This will change the treatment prognosis.

Injuries can happen ten, twenty or even thirty years before, and at the time will not seem like they were significant enough to cause any problems. The body is an amazing machine and can compensate for impact and misalignments for long periods of time before it says enough is enough.

With Emma we went through a series of treatments to take pressure off the neck and get rid of her headaches. But the main point is to retrace back to the likely cause of the issue, trying to repair that whiplash injury and make sure the headaches don't come back in the future.

Tom is a long-time client, in his early 50's and always brings his two lovely kids to our clinic. He has been working in the police for over twenty-five years, originally, what I thought was an active role, going out on patrol and keeping physically fit. He told me the opposite, it used to be like that at the start, but over the years he said, "I've become a paper pusher, in charge of larger teams, and for the last fifteen years have been sat behind a desk." This is one of the most common things we hear from our clients when they are struggling with back issues. Usually, a low back or a neck problem can be brought on from long-term sitting at a desk.

Tom was finding that he was fine in the mornings when getting in to work. His commute was forty-five minutes in the morning, and then he would sit down at his desk until 11am. He would then start to develop a tightness across the shoulders, tension in his neck, and become restless and fidgety.

He would need to get up and walk around, and his colleagues assumed he was going to the toilet.

He would take five minutes and stretch his back before coming back to begin another forty-five minute block of work. He would count the seconds to lunch break where he could go for a really long walk and stretch. In the afternoon, his low back would start to tense up and it then made it difficult to concentrate, as this was the most painful out of the two areas.

He had occupational health to perform a desk assessment, and he was given a new chair and the screen was put in the 'proper' position, so his desk was set up as good as it could have been.

Prolonged sitting is not good for our spines; it puts enormous pressure over a long period of time on the discs and facet joints (stabilising joints) in the spine and thus causes discomfort and often severe pain.

We started adjusting Tom's spine to get it in the best position and strengthened it up to prevent the issues coming back. We have to accept the fact that Tom always has to sit behind a desk for work; he has a family to provide for. But when we can get his spine in the best position it gives us the best chance of not letting the problem come back and allow him to work pain free.

Why do some people get pain and others don't?

Mrs Jones is a 43-year-old mother of two who works part time as an accountant in West Byfleet. She enjoys Pilates. On her two days off, she likes to take her dog for a walk and meet some girlfriends for coffee in Taylors. She also likes to keep fit in the gym, and when she's not doing Pilates, she enjoys a spin class. The summer is here and she's out playing tennis with many friends. The kids have lessons on the court next to her and enjoy a lovely glass of Pimms after the game. In the last few years she's been suffering with a lower back issue which always gets worse when she begins to play tennis in the summer months. Although this year, it is particularly bad, and it started affecting her tennis so much so she's had to start cancelling games with friends. She's realised that it wasn't necessarily the tennis that she loved, it was the social aspect and the fact that the whole family could get involved. Over the past three years, she's seen various physiotherapists, had massage, taken many forms of medication including naproxen, and also consulted with a spinal surgeon who took an MRI of her spine.

The MRI shows that she has an L5/S1 disc problem putting pressure on her spine. Tennis is a very dynamic sport and has lots of twisting and turning, this is why the disc has been flared up when she starts the tennis season. The disc is going out to the right-hand side therefore putting pressure on the right sciatic nerve, giving her a lightning rod pain going into her right buttock.

Mrs Jones has a friend called Mrs Williams. Mrs Williams has three kids, she works full time, and also enjoys Pilates with Mrs Jones. She sits at a desk all day and works as a PA for a corporate lawyer in the city. She barely finds time to get to the gym as much as Mrs Jones, and it's always on her mind that she's sitting for long periods of time during the day. She also has a back issue that is more consistent and not just seasonal depending on if she is doing more activity or not. She's conscious of it when she's sitting at a desk and has had numerous ergonomic assessments provided by her workplace. These have helped if the workload is high. On busy weeks, she is often in the office at eight o'clock and leaves at six some days, spending at least an hour on trains commuting backwards and forwards to London.

She has private medical health with her work and also has had an MRI. Believe it or not, she too has an L5/S1 disc issue. Without giving any confidential information away, it is very similar to Mrs Jones' disc problem.

They've both been around the block and seen many different people. Some things have helped, some haven't, but the underlying consensus is that nothing has fully resolved the problem.

Mrs Williams has a rare day off and invites Mrs Jones out for a walk and a coffee at Taylors. They bump into one of their other friends and get chatting about their backs. The friend in Taylors recommends them to see Dr Jeremy at West Chiropractic.

They make their appointments and are greeted by staff. Jeremy welcomes them into the clinic. An assessment with x-rays, posture analysis, and a full report is given and a detailed treatment program with a rehabilitation programme built in.

It gets to week three and everything is going well. Mrs Jones is feeling much looser and lighter. She has no sciatic pain and is able to get back to full time Pilates. But Mrs Williams still has buttock pain and still has back pain. I was wondering why she's not feeling like Mrs Jones? She has the same disc issue, the same level, the same symptoms, so why doesn't she respond the same?

This is all too common and highlights the importance that everybody is different. There is no one size fits all treatment program for lower back pain and disc issues. Discs can take anywhere from nine to twelve months to fully heal and it is largely dependent on how long they've had the problem for.

Pain affects everybody in different ways. One of the most common things we hear in the clinic is "When I'm stressed or had a long day, my back pain or shoulder pain is much worse." We will touch on this more when we discuss what causes back pain, but to make you aware there are not just structural issues causing pain within the spine. Many of our clients will describe an emotional trauma coupled with a physical trauma, for example a road traffic accident. It is often why a lot of spinal surgeries do not cause full resolution of spinal pain. What this means is you can take the pressure off the spine and still be left with pain.

We dug deeper into why Mrs Williams was taking longer to respond. After we looked at what she was doing outside of the clinic it became apparent that she wasn't looking after herself as well as Mrs Jones. She was making a couple of minor errors when she was getting home in the evening that were hampering her ability to heal at the rate that we wanted. The problem was how she was sitting at home and also how she was sleeping at night, we will talk more about this in the next chapter. But often we need to take a check at week 3 or 4 and see where we are with a progress evaluation, check the goals we set and perform a course correction. Like with an aeroplane, it never flies in a straight line as conditions are always variable, but minor course correction along the way ensures it gets to its final destination.

This also brings in the nature v nurture argument. We often hear "My mum has a really bad back and has done for years and so does her mum, so I was bound to have back pain." I can't sit here and argue with that, there is a genetic predisposition to back pain, but there is not much evidence out there, mainly because it is so hard to try and replicate the same conditions and the fact that back pain is so complicated.

Mrs Jones did say that she has a family history of back pain, but I have also seen clients that have had family members who have had major back operations and they have managed to avoid them with proper care and guidance.

The nurture of the human body and the way that it is influenced as we grow is more important than a nature or genetic aspect. I believe, with the proper guidance and care, that most genetic issues can be adapted and changed as we grow.

If there is a strong male lineage of disc issues on one side of the family, a long line of males performing manual and physical work, then I would look at this and say to my client "You have an opportunity to get your spine in the best position, so you can avoid going down the same route, keep working long term, and avoid surgery and maintain your independence." I never understand why some people work themselves into the ground with the mindset of "when I retire I will relax and get my back fixed". Often it is too late, the back has too much damage and the ceiling we can actually reach is much lower.

We work our whole lives to travel and 'enjoy' ourselves in retirement, but all too often our bodies can't keep up with the expectations of our mind and many of us don't end up travelling to Australia and climbing the Sydney Harbour Bridge or swimming on the Great Barrier Reef. The time was yesterday to get on top of your back, let alone any other health concerns. Treat your body like a race car, put the appropriate fuel in it and keep it tuned up.

On the argument of nature v nurture, we often see younger clients with scoliosis. This is an S-shaped curve in the spine which is most common in young females roughly around ten years of age, although it can be noticed later on in teenage years. Very often this can be a nature issue; the client is born with the curve and this can worsen over time. Usually this is discovered when the ribs start to rotate, and the child will notice tightness and discomfort or ill-fitting clothes.

A lot of medical doctors will monitor the curve and use brace techniques to try to minimise the impact as the child grows older. If the curve rises above forty degrees, then usually surgical intervention is deemed necessary, which puts two rods either side of the length of the spine to straighten it out. This often resolves the issue, but often we see many patients post-surgery who are still in pain and having headaches and back issues.

The spine can change and has been repeatedly shown by Chiropractic BioPhysics (CBP) and Dr Deed Harrison. It is the most researched technique in Chiropractic, and he has shown with pre and post x-rays changes in the spine over periods of time using non-surgical intervention. A study in 2017 on a 15-year-old female showed a reduction in scoliosis from twenty-seven degrees to eight degrees over a fifteen week period (Haggard *et al*, 2017).

The number one mistake with back pain

People always ask me for some of the things that I shouldn't be doing with my spine. It's probably become apparent now from reading this so far that there is no one size fits all answer for this question. Everybody's spine is completely different, and this will have a huge knock on effect on the advice that we give and the mistakes that people make. Before reading any further, always remember that it is best to get checked by a professional who can offer specific advice for your body rather than recommending a one size fits all program which may not yield positive results.

One of our clients called Mick was always asking advice regarding sleeping. Mick was 47 and had been a bricklayer his whole life. His body had been through a lot of physical stress. He was always finding that in the morning he was waking up with severe back pain, mainly across his shoulders going up into his neck. He thought it could be his pillows or his mattress, which he changed, but nothing happened. He bought one of those posture straps so that when he was working it would pull his spine backwards and take the pressure off his shoulders and neck.

We started by asking Mick what he was doing before bed. It turned out that he was lying on the sofa with his head turned to the side watching TV. This could be anywhere up to four hours. So, let me explain what is happening here: with the head turned to the left and the body staying straight, this puts a rotational stress through the neck and shoulders without Mick knowing it. Whilst he's lying there he isn't moving, therefore not changing the position, and the stress on the joints and discs in the neck builds up. He then gets up, feels fine and gets off to bed. The stress built up in the last four hours will dissipate through the neck and shoulders causing the muscles to tighten up, and therefore causing him to wake up with pain.

We also asked him about his sleeping position. He told me that he was sleeping with two feather pillows lying on his front with his head turned to the side. He had done this his whole life; it was the only comfortable position he could sleep in. In the past he had tried to sleep on his side or on his back, however, when lying on his side, it put more pressure through the side of the shoulder and he couldn't get comfortable. When lying on his back, he couldn't get a full night's sleep because his wife kept nudging him to stop him snoring. He remedied this by falling asleep in front of Match of the Day, but that wasn't a long-term solution due to tension in the marriage. I told him to get back in the bed.

So, what did we advise?

Well, firstly, we wanted to reduce the stress building up on his neck in the evenings, so we altered the position he was lying in on the sofa to make it more square on and so the neck wasn't twisted. Truly, the best position to relax in the evenings will be sitting upright with the knees lower than the hips to reduce stress on the lower back, and also with the neck resting on the top of the chair. When this is not possible and you have to lie down, then it's important to prop the neck up to keep it in line with the shoulders and thoracic spine. With all this Mick still had pain in the mornings, so we took it one step further and gave him a neck traction wedge to lie on before he went to sleep. These are often called Dennerrolls and are moulded to the shape of the spine to open up the joints and restore the normal neck curve. This takes pressure off the shoulders and the neck. For Mick, this was key before he got into bed. He lay on it for five minutes to begin with and gradually built it up to fifteen minutes until one time he told me he fell asleep on it because it became so comfortable. Obviously, I would not advise this for anybody, but it is a good sign as it means the neck shape has adapted to the wedge, and restoring the curve is the key to good spinal health and reducing pain.

(You can get a neck wedge from us, otherwise you can find them on Amazon. With everything it is best to have them custom fitted to provide the best results, which we do off the back of a posture assessment and often x-rays so we can see exactly which wedge is best.)

The next thing we did was address the pillows and sleeping position for Mick. It's best to use a uniform size pillow not a feather one, as they can change overtime and are also different every single night depending on which position you're in. So, an orthopaedic pillow is always good; probably not the one with the curves in it, as we found that they can be Marmite. What I mean by that is some people love them, some people hate them. There are great orthopaedic pillows on the market, rectangular and between ten and fifteen centimetres in depth, providing a uniform platform for the neck to rest on each night when sleeping. This means that every night Mick got into bed he was guaranteed to have the same position for his neck to be in.

There is now the issue of lying on the front with the neck twisted to one side. We rolled up a towel and put this between Mick's legs when he was lying on his side, which meant that he wasn't able to twist around onto his front or onto his back (for fear of a right hook in the face). Now obviously, at the start this was a difficult position to adapt to because he had spent the last forty plus years in that position. But what he did find is that because the neck was propped up it took pressure off the shoulders. After developing a good bedtime routine of neck stretching, the pain in the mornings began to ease as the neck came back into a better position.

He asked me, "Do I have to use this neck wedge forever?" I told him he didn't, which he was happy to hear, but physiological change remains in the body after nine to twelve months, and this is the same for anything. For any sort of marathon training or gym training, to see a physiological change can take anywhere up to a year. After his initial phase of care, which was two to three months, I recommended he used the wedge twice a week to maintain it up to the year mark.

Remember, it takes 28 days to build a habit!

Our next client is Kate. She is 63, mother of two, grandmother of five. Kate is amazing. She is one of the fittest 63-year-olds that I know and works full time. However, she does suffer from a chronic back issue which has been going on since she had her kids forty years ago. This is an all too common occurrence that many ladies tell me when they come to the clinic. There are two groups: ladies in their 30s and 40s who've just had kids that are one or two years old and found that throughout their pregnancies and when the babies were little, they developed back neck issues. The other group are in their 50s and 60s and have had back issues for the last twenty to thirty years that started after having kids.

For the first group, the young mums carrying a child is an incredibly stressful time emotionally but also physically on the body. In the third trimester the body releases a hormone called relaxin to allow the pelvis to expand during labour to allow the birth of the baby. This presents problems, as the baby grows in utero it puts more stress through the pelvis, which due to the relaxin is more malleable and can cause more pain. One of the most common pelvic issues in pregnancy is symphysis pubis dysfunction (SPD) where the pelvis becomes so loose that the front joint begins to rub and becomes inflamed causing immense pain when the mother walks.

After birth, the mother's pelvis is obviously moved in a different position. She has very little time to get anything sorted let alone do any home exercises to strengthen her pelvis. She's doing a great job caring for the baby. Overtime, that baby only goes one way weight wise, and that is up. As the baby gets heavier, the demands through the mother's body increase and the already problematic pelvis begins to present again. This is a cycle that can carry on for a number of years depending on how many children the mother has.

The pelvis doesn't return to normal and then the mother falls into category two, and twenty-thirty years later the pain becomes so bad that enough is enough. "Doctor Jeremy please help, my back pain started after my kids. Eighteen years of lifting them up, running around after them and ferrying them in the car has taken its toll, please help!" It was only when I first had my son I realised what mothers have to go through day to day, always putting the kids before them; mothers you are amazing! But you must look after yourself to be able to look after others. Don't leave it too long and don't suffer until the kids leave home.

So back to Kate, I got side-tracked. Kate is one of these mothers that had pain after her kids and left it. Now, thirty years later, she has decided to get something fixed. I asked her what she used to do to get rid of the back pain when it came on? She told me she would take painkillers and lie in bed for five days until it went away.

The episodes at the start would happen once a year and she would be laid up for almost a week. However, in the past ten years, the episodes are happening every three months more intensely and even lying in bed wouldn't fix the issue.

This brings me back to the title of the chapter: "The Biggest Mistake'! This is one of the old treatment methods for back pain back in the 50s and 60s. Patients were told by GPs to go home and put a hot water bottle on it while staying in bed until the pain resolved. We now know this is not effective anymore.

When Kate has back pain, her back will go into full spasm, and it will pull her hip up on the right side. She won't be able to straighten her back and will be walking (in her words) like the Hunchback of Notre Dame. Let me explain what is happening here, the body is incredibly clever and by putting the back muscles into spasm it is protecting the spinal cord and the discs from any damage. If Kate tries to move too far, therefore putting pressure on a disc or causing the disc to herniate, the muscle tightens up, causing pain and acting as a warning signal to not go any further.

The caveat: if you lie in bed for too long the muscles get stiffer, no blood gets to the area and it takes longer to recover. The muscles need to move, they need to have oxygen and vitamins going through them to reduce the spasm. Not immediately, but it does have to happen gradually. Therefore, gentle movements are the best way to reduce back pain in the short term.

I myself have suffered with back issues in the past and have recurring L5/S1 discs. Before I knew about Chiropractic and good spinal health my back would go into full spasm, and I too would rest in bed for two days at a time before things were back to normal, until I was told to keep moving, to which I muttered many expletives towards the person that recommended this.

The first few steps getting out of bed in the morning would be like no other pain, lightning bolts in the back shooting into the buttocks bringing tears to my eyes. Honestly, I have not had a pain like it; you wouldn't wish it on your worst enemy, and this is one of the reasons lower back pain is one of the main causes of disability worldwide.

I took the advice and kept moving with small steps around the house on one level, but no stairs just yet. As the hours went on, I would get more flexible and more mobile, and the hardness and swelling in the muscles would gradually reduce. And then in the evening the pain would dissipate, and I was back almost to full function. It's important to remember that there's still a lot of inflammation and swelling in the spine which is there for a reason, to protect the disc and nerves. So, going back to running, sitting for long periods or going to the gym was always a bad idea.

When I told this story to Kate, she thought I was crazy, and although she hasn't had any severe back spasms since being under Chiropractic care, she gets the odd niggle after gardening or the gym, but rather than resting with her feet up she carries on moving and ensures it doesn't develop into the old back spasms she used to have.

You may be reading this thinking there's absolutely no way I can move when my back is bad. I hear you; I was there, but even small movements just to get you out of the bed will make a huge difference in the recovery from a back spasm.

Why does it always come back

What if all these things are done? What if everything is put in place to ensure that the back pain doesn't come back? What if the core is the strongest it's ever been? The disc pressure has come off and the pelvis is looking strong as well. However, there is still pain, not as much but sometimes there can be a niggle or something that is causing an issue whilst gardening or picking up the kids.

We have to go back to the causes of back pain, look at the structural, chemical and emotional components to how it develops. Most of the examples we have spoken about so far have focused on the structural side of care, this is really important. For 90% of cases it will cause resolution when we get to the root cause of the issue. For that last 10% we must look deeper.

Chemical stress is what we are putting in our body and how it's interacting with our health. The most common type of toxic stress is smoking and alcohol. Obviously, they cause a lot of reactions throughout the body and will change the composition of certain tissues. If these tissues are already inflamed it only exacerbates the problem and will delay healing.

So how does that even work? You're telling me that when I drink alcohol it will make my back pain worse? There's one main element with alcohol stress on the body, with that being the fact that it dehydrates the patient, causing the tissues to become a lot tighter. If you think about wet towels and you begin to suck the water out of it, it becomes dry and fluffy. A similar thing happens to the tissues surrounding the spine. They are supposed to be holding the spine in place and able to move and adapt to the demands the body is putting on it. When they are dry and brittle, the discs will take up more stress and can cause back issues.

How does smoking work? Smoking has an impact on the body. When you breathe in from the cigarette, it causes the chemicals in cigarettes to be absorbed into the bloodstream which then goes around the body. These chemicals cause a free radical reaction, essentially where they have a mind of their own and run around and bounce off different cells in the body. When they go past an area that is damaged or inflamed it can exacerbate the issue. Picture this: a china shop with two damaged plates, and the lady who owns the shop is beginning to clean up the plates when two toddlers run into the store, hyped up on green smarties. They begin bumping into everything and causing more plates to smash and more damage. This is a similar way that free radicals from cigarettes work, they cause already damaged cells to become weaker and this then delays healing long-term. This is why when you break a bone, the doctor will recommend that you don't smoke as they have shown that smoking affects bone healing.

Other types of chemical stress include prescription medications. They put enormous amounts of stress on the body. One of the most common medications that is used is Ibuprofen or Nurofen (trade name). This is an anti-inflammatory or NSAID and works on the body to reduce inflammation. Well, hold on a second, if this drug reduces inflammation then surely that's a good thing? Yes, I see where you're coming from, however, the knock-on effect of an NSAID is that it reduces the mucus lining in the stomach. The stomach has lots of acid to break down food so that it can be absorbed further down the digestive tract. When you lose the thick padded lining of the stomach, it leaves it susceptible to damage from the acid and this can cause hernias over the long-term, which is where there is a hole in the stomach. This can cause major problems and can often result in surgery, which is not where we want to be.

There is always a time and a place for medications. I have seen my clients walk into me on crutches bent over at ninety degrees and not able to function. To get in the car they had to take some sort of pain medication, otherwise it wasn't possible. Pain medication such as Ibuprofen, Naproxen or Co-Codamol do provide short term relief, however, they shouldn't be used long-term to manage pain as they can cause worse side effects and compensations in the rest of the body.

I would always recommend when taking any sort of pain medication to use it with food and with a lot of water to limit the knock-on effect it has on the digestive system and the rest of the body. It's not my role to recommend when it is appropriate or not to be taking medication; this is a conversation to be had with a GP. With pain medications such as ibuprofen and naproxen, people do become over reliant on them and use them each day. The pain feels good when taking medication, and it's difficult to come off that when there is still an issue there putting pressure and causing pain.

The NSAID category such as ibuprofen and naproxen are anti-inflammatory drugs, and these are the ones that can damage to the stomach. Opioid medications such as co-codamol can block pain pathways with over-use of these for long periods of time, and the patient can risk becoming addicted much more commonly than taking NSAIDs. Non-opioid medication including paracetamol are one of the safer medications to take as they are less addictive and cause less issues with the stomach and digestive tract. It is still a stress for the body to process and can cause toxic stress on the liver.

Hope is not lost as there are some natural anti-inflammatories that can be administered and provide really good pain relief without having any side effects on the rest of the body.

Ginger, in its root and raw form, is one of the most powerful natural anti-inflammatories out there, and it can be taken in a juice or a smoothie or a tea. It's also in a supplement form, which isn't as effective and is not a natural source. The downside is that you have to have a lot of ginger to have the same effect as taking an ibuprofen.

Turmeric is also a great root vegetable that will provide a similar effect to ginger and can be taken in the same way either in a juice or a tea.

Omega 3 is a compound that is found in fats, more specifically oily fish and certain nuts like sunflower seeds and pine nuts. It works very similarly to an anti-inflammatory drug and has various other health benefits. What does oily fish mean? This is salmon, sardines, kippers and mackerel. There is absolutely no chance that I'm eating those and definitely not three times a week.

This is something that I would recommend is supplemented, as some of our patients do find it difficult to get three portions of oily fish into their diets each week. You can get a good quality omega 3 supplement from cytoplan.com for around £15, if you wanted to go to more of the Ferrari equivalent you can look at purebio.co.uk. It is a better-quality supplement, but if you are just starting out then it depends what your goal is. You can always email me at info@westchiropractic.co.uk, and I can provide some guidance.

There are plenty of other food items that can cause inflammatory effects on the body such as sugar and acidic foods. Foods that tend to be packaged or prepared will also have high numbers of artificial nutrition in them, which can cause the body to become inflamed and influence back pain.

So, you are telling me that if I'm eating chocolate and caffeine that will affect my back? This is a difficult concept to understand but I will try and make it as easy as possible. Firstly, with caffeine it is a dehydrant meaning it will draw water out of the body, which is why when you've had a lot of caffeine you feel very thirsty and your body is dehydrated. If you have a muscle spasm or a disc issue, then the water is sucked out the muscles causing them to be very hard and inflexible. The disc is 85% water, so there's less water in the body and it'll be reduced in size, causing more pressure in those areas.

Whether it's artificial foods such as sugar and artificial flavourings, they will affect the acid/alkaline balance of the body. If I take you back to chemistry (which I must be honest wasn't my favourite science), if you remember the pH scale and something that is a high pH is very alkaline and something that is a low pH is acidic.

The pH of the body is just over seven, and when this pH is maintained, most of its systems function in harmony. If the pH goes up to more of an alkaline balance, then a lot of research suggests that this is actually a good thing and is where a lot of nutritionists will try and get their clients. Many cancer patients will be on an alkaline diet as the theory suggests that the cancer cells cannot survive at a higher alkaline pH.

When we eat something acidic, bringing the pH lower, the blood will become more acidic and this is not good for cells and tissues in the body. Some foods that are very acidic like sugar, meat, processed foods and caffeine sustain a low pH for long periods of time can cause chemical disruption in the body and affect the ability of the body to heal.

The alkaline diet is very simple. The main concept is lots of raw, green leafy veg and a minimum amount of meat. Protein is sourced from nuts, seeds and eggs. There is very little processed food, and generally, if you're making most things from scratch, then your body is going to be in a more alkaline state.

So, we also have another stress on the other side of the triangle called Emotional Stress. This is best described after a long week of work, when you come home and the house is a tip, kids are running around and you are getting the dinner ready. You start to feel your shoulders tighten up and go into the neck, and you feel this sudden surge come around the head and develop into a tension headache. What happened? This is a primary emotional stress causing the body to have a physiological response to either move away from the stress and do something different or to try and relax. A lot of people, particularly after a long day at work, will use alcohol to wind down the body and reduce emotional stress. This works as the alcohol has a relaxing effect, but it's not a long-term coping method. You often find that people who start drinking on Friday after a long week but who do not drink on the Thursday after a long day, gradually creeps up the week until one glass of wine every night is not only having minimal effect on the emotional stress but also providing chemical stress to your body.

There are often more traumatic incidents as well such as relationship issues, bereavement, and accidents such as car crashes. These cause huge emotional stress on the body, and even though we cannot feel it or see it, it is still a huge amount of stress for the body to cope with. This must be managed by the body, and studies have shown that when we are stressed it causes a physiological response in the cells. Different hormones are released and the chemical composition of the blood and cells changes. If this is sustained long-term, it can cause adrenal stress and often burnout.

I talk to many people who work long hours and have busy lives, rushing here there and everywhere, myself included. It's only when you stop and take a check that you think *I can't sustain this long term*. It causes a huge drain on the body. I read an article the other day about partners at the 'Big 4' accountancy firms having a reduced life expectancy once retiring as the body is in constant fight and flight mode for forty years of working. Minimal sleep, poor diet, high stress and high stress from toxins. As things in the body start to break down, we seek medical advice and take pill after pill, all the while piling up this toxic and emotional stress on the body.

Where my clinic is positioned, we see a lot of our patients who work in the city with busy jobs and busy lives. Commuting each day is draining and also puts your body in a state of mind that can result in stress overload.

So how does emotional stress cause back issues? It's not that a negative emotion will go to your back and say "I've had a rubbish day, you are going to hurt now." It affects your body's ability to deal with pain. So, very often, the body can block out or compensate for an issue in the spine by recruiting other muscles or walking differently. When there is emotional stress that is an emergency, it must deal with this first before trying to deal with the pain issue. And it brings it to the surface much more quickly and apparently (Yin, 2001).

We have a client who I will call Emma, she is twenty-six and works extremely hard for a company in London. She is up early to 'get a seat' on the train at Woking. As a side note, she says to me "I pay all this money, I'm not standing", to which I do agree.

Anyway, she has been seeing us on and off for six years, and we can always trace her problem to an emotional issue. Well, how do I know?

We do all of our normal work, locate the root cause of her structural issue, which clears up after a matter of sessions, and Emma begins to function better; headaches subside and jaw relaxes off (remember I said the jaw is really important for headaches). But we will still see her coming back after four-six weeks with the same thing. I do all of my testing again, clear it all out, and the same pattern reappears.

So, when we see things coming back we have to ask ourselves, hold on, what else is going on here? With Emma I started asking her, how do you sleep? What do you do outside of work? What do you eat? How do you relax in the evening? None of which were arousing any suspicion of a problem.

I began to ask her what work was like, to which she told me it was awful. High stress environment, boss always on her back and other colleagues bickering and gossiping about each other. Office politics but to another level it seemed.

I began to ask her about how she felt when this was going on, about how it made her body react when her boss was causing her to be upset. Over the next few weeks, she began to see a pattern. Whenever there was a high stress situation in the office she would become tense and could feel her neck and jaw tightening up. She would begin to grind her teeth. When this happens, Emma always knows that she is going to suffer with a headache.

So, we could trace the headaches back to the stress at work, but how could we change that? We can't just keep treating her, as it's not getting to the root cause of the issue. I recommended some Headspace techniques she could do on the train to try and re-train her emotional reaction to stressful situations. The problem is we can't take our patients out of these situations at home or work. It's about changing the body to better cope with the problem.

This helped Emma and she found that she didn't tense up as much. However, it ultimately meant that she had to leave this role, mainly due to the pain she was getting, but also no one wants to be treated the way she was, and she deserved better. I'm happy to report she is now doing really well. She still gets the occasional headache but it's not due to her work situation and is managed with exercise and adjustments here at the clinic.

I have seen traumatic episodes such as car accidents causing PTSD that have a knock-on effect for years after and see patients in head to toe pain because of it. No rhyme or reason why the pain is there, as in there is no structural component when we examine and x-ray. But chronic and debilitating pain. Often, when the doctors can't see anything wrong on the scans or MRI's, there is a blanket term labelled to global pain patients called fibromyalgia. It is an arthritic syndrome causing pain all over the body. Often this can be traced to an emotional stress. A relationship breaking down, losing a job, or traffic accident.

When this is the case and we can build a good relationship with the patient, it is often that I would recommend seeking some professional psychological help to work through the trauma induced by these stresses. We would work as a clinical team to help reduce the overall symptoms of the body, us from a structural point of view and the psychotherapist from an emotional side.

How to resolve back pain

So, we have talked about what causes back pain and how it is different for everyone. This next part must be the easy bit, right? There must be this magic solution that will get rid of back pain.

All too often this is what we hear. I wish this were the case and we could click our fingers and wipe the back pain away. Unfortunately, it's just not the case. As complicated as back pain is to understand, it is also equally as complicated to get rid of. Different techniques work well on others and some do not work at all on some clients.

What is a guarantee is that as practitioners we learn a wide variety of techniques and can alter treatment plans depending on how someone is responding. The longer a condition has been going on for then usually (not always) the longer it takes to fix.

We will talk about the methods we use with our clients in this chapter and why some work better than others. The first section will be simple daily habits that can be adjusted as soon as you put this book down, the next section will be more in-depth exercise rehabilitation that will take time to learn and become accustomed to. The second section may require us to tailor the exercises to you. If this is the case, please email me at info@westchiropractic.co.uk or call me on 01932 355529.

Sitting

What is something that a large majority of the population do daily for a large proportion of the day? SITTING! We all sit for too long. If you look back to our ancestors, the cavemen had huge back muscles and big gluteal muscles keeping them upright. We were not designed to be sitting crouched over flexed all day, some people for at least eight hours per day. Over time, this causes an evolution of the body, our shoulders will become rounded, our back weak, and our head will shoot forward.

There are studies being written about how the average 9-5 worker will change their body shape drastically in the future. This has huge consequences for how the body will function. The rib cage provides support and protection for the heart and lungs. If the ribcage begins to tilt forwards and the head goes following suit, this will put compression on the heart and lungs and could affect their function. If the heart is having to work harder to pump blood around the body and the lungs are having to force air through a compressed rib cage, this will cause them to wear out quicker. My prediction could be an increase in cardiovascular and respiratory issues due to the changing physiology of our bodies.

Not to mention the stress on the spinal cord. If you think of a long elastic band going down from your head all the way to the bottom of your spine, if the head starts to move forwards, it will stretch the spinal cord and put stress through that. The spinal cord is the lifeline between the brain and the rest of the body, so it's vital this is kept intact.

They say that sitting is the new smoking. Don't get me wrong, I think long-term smoking is also bad and detrimental for your health, but what will cause the biggest change in your back pain is the position we sit in and how we position our bodies throughout the day. So many people sit for work and they say to me, "There is no way I can stop sitting, I can't concentrate if I'm not sitting for work behind my computer."

But why is sitting so bad?

The low back was never designed to be in a sustained position for long periods of time. The muscles either side of our spine are called the erector spinae; they keep us erect or upright. They aren't there to hold everything together when we are sitting. The disc at the base of the spine is also vital to keeping healthy when we sit. Think of a jam donut, not one of those ones from Greggs but a big plumpy and doughy donut. That is what your bottom disc looks like (minus the sugar coating). When we sit, this takes up the majority of the load. This disc's purpose is to distribute the load and also act as a cushion between the bones, but not for long periods of time. This is why office workers who don't practice proper spinal hygiene often develop low back disc issues.

So the remedy must be don't sit? Well not quite. As we have mentioned, a lot of people must sit for work. So how do we get the body in the optimum position to sit in?

Firstly, the knees need to be lower than the hips. This takes pressure off the low back and allows the force from the shoulders and head to be distributed evenly through the pelvis rather than the low back. The elbows should be tucked into the sides, the chin tucked back and the shoulder blades pinching together. When first starting to do this, it is very unlikely that you can sustain the position for longer than around ten minutes before something starts to feel achy or even painful. So have a post-it note on the desktop which reminds you to assume the position. You could do ten minutes on and then ten minutes rest, repeating this throughout the day.

We do desk assessments, so if you want us to visit your office and do a desk assessment for you and your colleagues, then look at our website www.westchiropractic.co.uk, and we can book it in. As a side note we also do wellness talks for local companies and community groups, check out www.drjeremyspeaks.co.uk

Another way to reduce the stress on your back is to stand up. Completely reset the spine and walk around for two minutes and allow the muscles to stretch out. There is a concept called creep. If you think about putting consistent pressure on the jam donut over eight hours, then it is gradually going to compress and more jam will be pushing on the sides of the doughnut. If you take the pressure off, then suddenly, the dough springs back up and resets. This is the same concept for your low back and the discs. We recommend taking all phone calls standing up.

But what about a standing desk? If your workspace has the capability and you have won the battle with HR to get a standing desk, then I would highly recommend it. They are becoming common in the workplace and are providing huge benefits to a lot of people. I would recommend starting off with fifteen-minutes of standing and then sit down for forty-five minutes. Then gradually alter the ratios until you are standing for much of the day. This trains the gluteal muscles to become active and much stronger, which will provide a lot of support to the base of the spine. Not only are you preventing back issues but training a muscle to give it support for that evening run or weekend tennis match.

Sleep Position

This is always a difficult one to remedy. "I can't control myself when I'm asleep, I'm asleep Doc." I always laugh as it's true, but we can put some measures in place to ensure that when we are asleep our body stays in a reasonably similar position as we started.

Why would sleeping be bad for our backs? Same as sitting, in that we are adopting a position for a long period of time. For some (should be for most), it is eight hours or more of lying down. So, if you are curled up like a pretzel, that is a long time to have that much stress on your body. If you are in a good position, this can be a really good time for your spine to breathe and relax and set you up for the day.

The main three positions people sleep in are on your back, front, and side. The front is the worst position as, generally, an arm will be up and the head tilted to the side. This causes the neck to rotate and will put pressure through the upper back. Then if you go and sit down for eight hours in the day, this puts you at risk of neck and shoulder issues.

The middle one is sleeping on the back. A good position, as the spine is aligned and the head is propped up by a pillow. But you do risk getting thumped by the person next to you for snoring.

So the best position? You guessed it right, the side. The side with the arms in front of you, head and hips in line with the legs at forty-five degrees, knees coming up to chest. This keeps the low back curve maintained at forty degrees and the rest of the spinal curves maintained.

Common Troubleshooting:

"I can't lie on my side as my shoulder hurts." This is common and often due to the shape or height of the pillow, which we will talk about further down.

"I start on my side and then end up on my front." The way to remedy this is to use a pillow or rolled up towel between the legs at the knee, and this will prevent the body from rolling around at night. It will feel strange at first, but your body will get used to it.

"I've always slept on my front; I can't break the habit." I agree. Once a habit is formed it is hard to break. We are not expecting miracles over-night and for you to wake up in the morning with no pain. Be kind to yourself. It may take weeks or even months, but keep starting on your side and gradually your body will adapt. Even if you are waking up on your front, the aim is to get more time on the side.

Mattress and Pillows

This leads us on to which is best? I used to recommend a mattress and pillow religiously because that is what the research said was best, and I didn't care what anybody at Memory Foam or Tempur said. The research knew best. What I did find as I recommended this mattress is that it wasn't right for everyone and people would come back saying that "I've had the worst night sleep." The first bit of advice would be to always buy a mattress with a ninety-day guarantee so you can send it back. A mattress needs to support you but not be so firm that you bounce off when you lie on it. I would look at a 4 on the scale and something that is pocket sprung orthopaedic. The problem with memory foam is that, although it is super comfortable, it does not give you as much support. If you already have a spinal issue, then the memory foam won't prop the back up, it will allow it to sink down, and this then causes the spinal curves to become distorted. Over time, if you are spending eight hours of your day like this, it gradually allows the spine to take its own shape.

With a firmer orthopaedic mattress, it may feel uncomfortable at first, but longer term, you will reap the rewards of better spine health.

Which pillow is best? The problem with pillows is that the feather ones aren't uniform, so one night you may get a good chunk of pillow and your head will be propped up and not in line with the rest of your body and you wake up with neck pain. The next night you may find you haven't much of the pillow, and this will force the neck the other way and cause a neck issue.

Pillows are one of the easiest things to change when it comes to back and neck pain, although some of my clients have told me they have tried every single pillow on the market. Some range from £20 to £200. If you are going to spend a lot of money on one, then the same advice as for the mattress. Make sure there is some sort of guarantee and you can take it back or swap it. I recommend a harder and more solid pillow that provides support through the spine and will be the same night after night.

You can find an orthopaedic pillow that has ridges on it, but they tend to be a bit harder to get used to. I would start with an orthopaedic uniform pillow; https://thebamboopillow.co.uk/ have a great one, and it's not going to break the bank.

Ice v Heat

One of the most common questions we get asked is, "should I use ice or heat?" And my response often surprises people. The research would suggest that for an acute injury (anything less than three months old) then you should use an ice pack. Anything longer would be classed as chronic and heat should be used. I have a different opinion, in that if you have a back injury, take a swollen disc for example, that has been grumbling away for the last three years on and off, and it has flared up, you don't want to be putting heat on what would be classed as a chronic issue. The reason being the disc is like a 'jam donut'. What happens when you heat up a jam donut? It gets all gooey and the jam begins to press on the sides of the dough.

Same thing happens here. When you begin to put heat on the spine, it will feel good for a short period of time and you will get more oxygen and blood to the area, but over the course of a day or even week, if this carries on then it is causing the disc to become more and more inflamed and affecting the ability for it to heal. It feels great while the heat is on, but as soon as it comes off, then it brings back the problem.

So, the alternative is to put ice on the area. What does ice do? Well, putting an ice pack on a recently sprained joint or inflamed area will reduce inflammation. What I mean by inflammation is swelling and fluid. Now, in the spine this is good after an acute injury, as it essentially acts as an airbag to protect all the integral structures like the disc and spinal nerves. However, as it goes on long term, it causes stiffness and mobility issues. So, putting ice on an acute injury will reduce the inflammation slowly.

But putting ice on a more chronic issue, something that has been going on for months and years, is also more beneficial as it will reduce any inflammation that is there. What I tend to advise is that if a patient has had a flare up, then to put heat on first for ten minutes then use an ice pack for ten minutes and repeat the process over an hour.

Do frozen chicken breasts count as ice? The short answer is yes, it works but it's probably not the most practical thing to use. You can get yourself a reusable ice pack on amazon, or frozen peas work well, as they mould to the shape of the spine. As far as heat goes, the wheat bags are great as you can put them in the microwave and they will give you ten minutes of heat, or a hot water bottle.

Pilates and Yoga

"Which is best? I'm not into that hippy yoga, do I really need to do it?" Okay, let me try and give my breakdown and experience with both modalities. Please remember, I'm not trained in either of these but will try and give my opinion from a chiropractic perspective (if you want to find out more about Yoga head over to our podcast or Youtube channel to watch an interview with Becca Sullivan who is a Yoga teacher).

Yoga has many of its origins from Eastern culture and has a spiritual attachment to it. There are many teachers that will steer clear of this approach but also many that will build a lot of spiritual work into their classes. It all depends what you are looking for. There are many different types of yoga, and from talking with Becca and various yoga teachers, if you are starting out, then a Hatha class seems to be one of the more popular ones.

With back pain and starting yoga it's important to remember you will be stretching a lot, and many sustained stretches over long periods of time, often two-three minutes. Number one must do, is to inform the instructor of your back issue. Most will be able to know what is good for your spine and what is not, and they can modify certain moves for you.

For example, if you are attending a yoga class and have a neck issue, then performing anything on your head is a bad place to start, or if you have a low back issue then doing seated reach forward with your chest compressing your spine is also not going to be beneficial long-term.

The sustained stretching is good for the spine as it will bend it and flex it as it was designed to. It adds an extra layer of flexibility back to the ligament and muscles and can reduce pain. I would be careful when doing rotation stretching; twisting too much can put pressure on discs and should be done carefully. Personally, I'm a fan of yoga. I believe, when done with a cautious instructor who has experience with people who are recovering from back injuries, then it can have a beneficial effect and prevent recurrence. I also enjoy the breathing, and it relieves emotional stress, which is beneficial for you and, as you will read, emotional stress can impact our pain as well.

Pilates was developed more recently in the 1920s by Joseph Pilates (Sorosky *et al*, 2007). He originally designed it in a hospital with springs and bands to rehabilitate patients. He got such fantastic results that he developed the practice. Originally, he built the system around his patients using the reformer machine, which if you haven't seen it, it's a sliding carriage with a padded surface that moves with springs under different tension depending on which you want to use. This was the beginner starting point, and then his patients would develop and build towards the mat-work, or what most of us commonly associate with Pilates. So many of us, myself included, started Pilates on the mat. Why is this if this is the most advanced method? Well ease and practicality are the main ones. It's costly and difficult to get twenty people on a reformer machine.

It is much more practical buying twenty mats and renting a room or a gym and doing it that way. Obviously, this can present issues in the ability to identify certain feelings like, tightening of the core, activating the pelvic floor or glutes. These are all vitally important techniques to be able to do to ensure you get the most out of a Pilates class.

I find Pilates to be incredibly effective when done properly with the proper guidance. Same rules apply as for yoga; make sure the instructor knows what is going on with your back, and they can modify it for any moves.

Pilates will strengthen rather than lengthen as yoga does. Although there is stretching in Pilates classes, the main focus is to strengthen the core and pelvic floor areas. This is why it is a great practice for mothers returning from pregnancies. A strong core and glutes is fundamental to ensuring we have a stable spine; they will act as a natural brace around the back, holding it in position. When we have a strong core brace, it means that movements like bending down, getting out of the car or picking kids up have much less of a chance of putting pressure through the spine and causing any back spasm.

The stronger you are, the less likely you are to have long-term issues with the back. If you had to push me for my preference, it is Pilates. I have done more of it and tend to get more benefit from it. But as you will read in this book, there is no right or wrong for one person. What works for you may not work for somebody else who is displaying exactly the same symptoms.

Brace

"Using a back brace really feels comfortable."

Yes, I completely understand that it feels great. Your back is in place and you can bend and move all around. Why wouldn't you wear one the whole time?

Look at professional weightlifters, they always wear a back brace when they go heavy to keep their spine in good shape. I know we are looking at the other end of the scale and you are not looking to clean and jerk 200kg tomorrow (maybe next week?).

But the same concept applies in that the purpose of the brace is to hold the spine in the best position, so it does the job the core and glutes should be doing.

This follows on really well from the Pilates section above, in that Pilates will get the core strong and hold the integral structures in place in the spine. It could be said that a lot of spinal issues can develop from poor control in the core, from sitting for too long or too much inactivity.

The brace will switch off the core and make it inactive. If this keeps happening over long periods of time, then it will become redundant, and you will feel you need to always use the brace to keep your spine in place. Same as a knee brace, it switches off all the muscles and ligaments around the knee that support it. This is no good when you don't have it on.

I do believe there is a time and a place for a back brace, for example, when moving house and having to lift boxes, doing gardening or when you have to lift something and there is no other way to do it. Put the brace on for extra support, but at all costs do not become reliant on it; it will cause more bad then good long term.

We stock them in the clinic. If you would like one, then text BRACE to +447588703680.

Wobble Cushion

These are really effective for use in the office or at home, as they distribute the weight evenly through the buttocks and legs. Not only that, but they also allow the spine to flex and move when you are sitting rather than being static. This nourishes the discs, as it allows them to move slowly and gently.

For roughly £10 this can save your spine. It won't be comfortable and will feel strange for the first few weeks, but gradually, you will get more and more used to it and will be thankful you bought one.

They need to be slightly squishy, so not pumped up the whole way, and you can rock from side to side and front and back, even diagonally. If it causes any issues, let me know, but pick one up off Amazon and give it a try for at least three weeks to notice the difference.

Desk Setup

If you work behind a desk more than twenty hours per week, then this section is vitally important for you. Even if you don't have pain when you are at your desk, it can affect your body's ability to heal. If the desk setup isn't designed with your spine in mind, then you aren't doing yourself any favours. A few simple tweaks can make a huge difference. Believe me, we have visited some of the big companies in the area and some of the ergonomic assessments have not been specified to the individual and it has caused serious problems.

The first aspect to check is the screen height, the top of the screen needs to be just above eye level. Best way to check all of this is with a side photo taken by a colleague, and you can check yourself or send to us and we will draw the lines and angles on for you and send it back with our recommendations.

The second point is the shape of the spine. Generally, we will see a curve in the spine and that the areas around the shoulder blades are too far back, so it will put pressure on the low back and cause the head to push forwards. Simply move the chair forwards or bring the keyboard closer and this will reduce the curve and allow the head to come backwards.

The third easy tweak is keeping the feet flat on the floor, with the knees lower than the hips and legs not crossed. If a patient is slouching and leaning back on a recliner it will generate more pressure on the base of the spine.

Footwear

The type of footwear is really important. Let's start with high heels. When walking in high heels it causes the pelvis to tip forwards and cause more of a curve in the base of the spine, putting pressure on the back. They tend to be worn in the evening for social events, where you have to stand for long periods of time or even dancing. This excessive pressure is not good for the spine. Always wear flat shoes where you can.

"Well what about flip-flops?" These are also not good; they cause the big toe to tighten up to hold on to the flip-flop to prevent it from falling off, this means the calf becomes tense, hamstring will then follow, and this pulls the pelvis out of shape, causing more issues in the spine.

Try wearing sandals with straps rather than a flip-flop. It's difficult whilst on holiday I know.

Have you seen the 'barefoot' shoes? These are the shoes that have very little sole. They are designed to allow the contours of the foot to mould around the surface you are walking or running on, bringing us back to our ancestors who used to walk around barefoot.

They are good but need to be used carefully. If someone was running 10k three times per week, you would consider them a serious runner. They wouldn't be able to switch to barefoot shoes and carry on running at this volume. It's a completely different running style and would need to be gradually built up. Some research suggests it can often take a full year to build up to your pre-barefoot intensity (Lieberman, 2012).

Exercise

"My doctor always tells me to go and exercise; lose weight and your back pain will go away."

The last thing you want to do when your back pain is bad is go out and exercise or go for a long walk. We mentioned earlier that going for a small walk or moving around the house is good when you have a back spasm, as the blood will flow more effectively to the back muscles and provide oxygen to reduce the spasm and take away the inflammation.

So which exercise should I be doing? Well, if you have had an acute back episode, then I would do as above, just gentle movement around the house, try lying on the floor and gently moving the knees from side to side or gentle rocking. You don't want to be moving too much when your back 'goes', the reason it has gone in to spasm is to keep everything in place.

Once the back spasm has reduced, then we can look at beginning to exercise again. To start with and to keep it as simple as possible, we want to start with anything low impact. The reason being that high impact activities like running or jumping will cause more shock and load to go through the joints and the back, when they aren't strong enough to be taking up this load. A gentle walk is the best place to start, even if it is just five minutes around the block. We can always build on this. Rome wasn't built in a day, and this is exactly the same concept that the 'couch to 5k' programme was built on. Small and achievable steps over a longer period of time rather than jumping up and going straight to the end. If you go to step 10 with your back straight away, you will end up on the floor again.

It's so important to listen to your body when recovering from a back injury. Even when you feel ok, it's key to remember where you were, as when the pain disappears there is still an issue there. We often see clients coming back two months later saying, "I did a half marathon this weekend" or "that gardening that needed doing, I couldn't resist, but feel it's put me back a few weeks."

Make sure when walking that you are wearing supportive footwear. High heels don't count (don't get me started on high heels). Trainers with a cushion on the bottom are good, a pair of running shoes like Asics work wonders. You don't need to break the bank; you can pick up a decent pair for around £50.

The important thing about the shoe is that it cushions when the heel touches the floor when walking so the back doesn't take up all the absorption of the strike. This is why a lot of people are wearing those 'minimal' or 'barefoot' shoes when running, as it forces you to land on your forefoot and minimises the load going through your spine. It's a great idea if people didn't think that completely changing their running and walking cycle would cause problems elsewhere, like shin splints, knee issues and strained calves. So it's really important to build it up super slowly if you do use something like that.

Start small and build gradually, pick a landmark like a pub or shop and factor this into your day, every day. Do it on the way to work or on a lunch break. Gradually, as your back begins to get used to this movement, we can then increase the length of the walk.

When can I run again? Usually at least a month after the last symptomatic episode. The reason being that there is no point going back to it when you are going to cause more damage. I'm writing this book at the time of the Covid-19 outbreak, and sorry to reference this, but it's a nice comparison. If we release the lockdown too early, there will be a surge in the number of cases, and we may have to go back into lockdown (according to the government). Same thing with physical activity, if we go back in, we may go back to square one.

What about the gym? The gym is a great place to build strength and core stability, but it's important to be doing the right things. We have some great links with personal trainers in the area who help our clients build long-term strength and prevent recurrence of their back pain. Email me on info@westchiropractic.co.uk, and I can send you their details.

With the gym, you don't want to be doing anything that causes your back to be painful. An ache or muscle soreness the day after is different. I'm talking sharp pain that feels different to the 'gym ache'.

Weightlifting when done correctly will support the back. I would not do any complex Olympic lifting without the supervision of an expert trainer. I'm also not a fan of the deadlift. Reason being the margin for error isn't worth it. The benefit of extra strength in the low back and hips is far outweighed by the damage it can do to your back. If you are just 1mm out or something is off when doing a deadlift, it can cause huge pressure through the disc. There are many other ways to build strength in the back that don't compromise it. We will touch on these further on.

Anything overhead, so overhead squatting, standing shoulder press and shoulder jerks should be avoided, as it's a quick movement that can put pressure on the low back.

If just starting out in the gym I would stick to machines. They give you a predictability of load and direction. Then, as you become more confident, move on to the free weights. These give a better recruitment and activation of different muscles around the joint. But be slow and controlled when doing them to activate the muscles properly.

Swimming is brilliant for backs and necks. It is non-load bearing, meaning there is minimal load going through the joints. You get in the water and feel weightless. This is great as it means your back discs and joints can rest whilst the muscles are worked and lubricated through a full range of movement.

It's not all that simple though (it never is unfortunately). It's important to be careful if you have any underlying knee or hip issues when kicking, particularly with breaststroke. It can put excess pressure on the hip, which can cause pain in the back as well. I recommend front crawl legs with breaststroke arms, to make things really confusing. But it's the best stroke, and also the one that will cause the least damage.

Front crawl is also good, but the torsion through the upper back when breathing can cause issues with neck pain. So just take care if recovering from neck pain with this one.

Exercises to get you out of pain - Stretching Exercises

These next set of exercises are great if you have recently injured your back. They will take pressure off the spine by stretching ligaments and muscles gently, allowing inflammation to be moved out of the muscles so you can become more mobile and gradually get back to normality. These won't correct the back issue, but they will act as SOS movements.

If you would like further information then you can get our report '12 ways to live with less back pain in 2 weeks' by texting '*back*' to **07588703680**

1. **Happy Cat/Angry Cat** - this is a great technique to mobilise the muscles either side of the spine from the low back all the way to the neck. You can do it first thing in the morning as soon as you get out of bed, or you can even do it in bed. A lot of our clients will find that they can't get out of bed in the morning, as it's the most painful then. This exercise allows you some flexibility and mobility to get up.

    You want to start on all fours, knees in line with the hips, and the shoulders stacked over the wrists. Slowly scoop the chin toward the chest so you are looking down and then raise the hips up, pushing the ribs up to form a C-shaped curve in the whole of the back, hold for three seconds and then go the other way. So, hips go forward, a curve starts in the low back and the head comes back. All the time breathing through these cycles and taking it really slow. You want to do it 10 times, and this should really take at least a minute, then repeat another 2 times.

    VIDEO LINK: https://youtu.be/KmTcyzfWluM

2. **Cross over stretch** - this is a great exercise for stretching the glutes. These are your bum muscles and provide all the stability and strength in the base

of the spine. When we stand up, walk or go up stairs, the glutes are the muscles that drive our torso up and through to allow the body to move through a gait cycle.

All too often, these muscles are weak and de-activated because we sit for too long, they become underutilised and will cause the back to become weaker. Like if a tent didn't have its guide ropes, it would still stand up, but it would be flapping around in the wind a lot more and be more likely to topple over if there was a big storm.

There are different versions of this exercise, but the first can be done when you are sitting in a chair. You cross the leg over the other knee and very gently pull the upper leg across your body until you feel a stretch in the bum muscle on that side. The pull of the muscle also stretches out some of the back fascia releasing off the stress placed on the back.

Hold the stretch for up to 30 seconds on both sides and remember not to bend forwards and compromise the spine when doing this seated.

The level 2 version of this exercise is lying down on your back. Again, crossing the leg over the opposite knee and then threading the hands through the hole you have created with that leg, pull the legs towards your chest, and you will feel the stretch in the glute on the crossed over leg side. Hold for 30 seconds or as long as you feel comfortable, no more than 30 seconds though. Repeat another 2 times on both sides.

VIDEO LINK: https://youtu.be/oiUFi_0CTSU

3. **Child's pose -** this is a great yoga stretch and is a really good transition exercise to move from one to the next. That is what it was originally used for in yoga classes, to keep the flow of the movements and allow the body to reset and get back in a good position. It lengthens the spine from head to tail, so it's good for low back and neck pain, but also, if you modify it to bring the chest further down to the floor, it's also really good for mid back pain. So great for office workers, drivers or anyone that sits for long periods of time.

Start on all fours, similar to number 2. You want to gently drop the arms in front of your palms (facing down) and slide them out away from your legs. Slowly drop the buttocks back so they are resting on top of the heels and gently feel the stretch through your back. You can push the buttocks back further to really feel the stretch in the base of the spine. If you drop the chest down even more, you will feel more of a stretch in the mid back. Keep the neck neutral and look down.

This is a sustained stretch so no longer than 30 seconds, repeat another 2 times through.

VIDEO LINK: https://youtu.be/H4Re33d3KUQ

4. **Wall Angel** - this is an exercise that we recommend to almost all of our clients as long as they don't have any shoulder issues. The reason being is that it does the complete opposite of what we all do every single day at work: sitting for too long. We have our shoulders and upper back rounded and our lower back in a flexed position, putting pressure through the base of the spine.

We were never designed to be in this position for an hour let alone eight or sometimes more. This exercise can be done throughout the day to reset the spine and take pressure off the upper back and help lengthen the lower back and relieve some stress on the discs.

If you don't mind the stares and odd looks from some of your work colleagues, I would do this every hour at work. Or sneak to the bathroom.

You need a wall to press against, so it needs to be fairly robust. Have the feet, shoulder width apart, bum touching the wall, then the arms up in a T-shape above the head at 90 degrees. You want to keep the head touching the wall and maintain all of these contact points throughout the exercise.

Slowly draw the low spine back so you are trying to flatten the curve in the base of the spine by drawing the abdomen in as well. If you are doing it correctly, you should feel it in the tummy and also across the shoulders and the shoulder blades.

You will want to hold this for 30 seconds at a time, repeating 3 times. In the morning, when you are waiting for the kettle to boil, start the first round, pour the water in, then let the tea brew during the second round, tea bag out and then let the tea cool, third round done.

VIDEO LINK: https://youtu.be/plijyJRVvTY

Exercises to make sure back pain doesn't return - Strengthening Exercises

Once the pain has subsided and normal function has resumed, then it's important we never go back to that stage. I suffer with a bad back and can empathise with my clients, that when it 'goes' it is agony. The pain for me doesn't initially hit me until later on in the day. If I do something in the gym or bend awkwardly then that is me finished for three days. The intensity builds over the day until one side will completely spasm up, and I will be bent over like the 'Hunchback of Notre Dame'. My back will gradually loosen off as the spasm reduces. I'm pleased to say that I have been working on my back a lot over the past three years and haven't suffered a spasm. I occasionally feel stiffness, but I do gym work and running so that niggle is inevitable. I have practiced these exercises we will go over now, regularly.

The most important thing to remember is that when the pain has gone, the problem has not gone. All too often we hear clients saying, "Oh, I feel pretty good now. I'm just going to go back to tennis and running". This is great as that was the original goal, and I'm so pleased they can do this. However, it's like an iceberg, the pain is always just the tip, and when clients rush back in without the symptoms to warn them when they are moving incorrectly, not warming up or building core strength around the injury, then it can reoccur. So, if you are at this stage now, I beg you, remind yourself what it was like when your back was bad and keep doing the exercises.

Only 15% of patients recovering from a musculo-skeletal injury will carry on the exercises past the four-week mark from their last appointment. To make a physiological change in the body it does take twenty-eight days, to sustain, it can take almost a year, depending on the nature and degree of the injury. It's so important to keep training and improving your back health.

The first three exercises here come from Professor McGill who is an expert in biomechanics. He has worked with professional athletes and many Olympic rowers to understand more about the biomechanics behind the spine, to try and improve function and movement. These exercises work for pro athletes and can work for us as well. They are very simple to implement and can be done on the living room floor as soon as today (McGill, 2015).

1. **Curl Up** - this is a modification of a sit up. A sit up is a major mistake a lot of our clients make. They are very bad for your spine in that they compress the bottom disc and put pressure through the base of the spine

when it is flexed over to bring the torso towards the knees. They have now been taken out of Marine training in the USA, as they were causing too many back issues. So if the Marines aren't doing them because they cause too many issues then we certainly can't do them (McGill, 2015).

The Curl Up is a safe alternative to a sit-up and doesn't flex the torso all the way over the base of the spine. It maintains the neutral spine and keeps the integrity in the discs whilst building strength in the core and transversus abdominis. This is the muscle that runs from the front of the tummy round into the back and pelvis. It acts like a brace but a natural one.

The exercise is started lying on your back, the hands by the side to start with. Slowly flex the knees and draw the heels towards the buttocks and keep them at 45 degrees. The next step is to put the hands underneath the back in the low spine where there is a gap. You should feel the gap reduce when the exercise is initiated, and this will mean you have complete core contraction.

Very slowly, whilst keeping the neck in a neutral position (not jutting the chin out, or looking all the way up), you want to bring the shoulders and head off the floor, feeling the contraction of the lower abdomen and tummy muscles. Keep this contraction going as you slowly lower the shoulders and head down to the floor.

Rest the neck down, contract the abdomen and raise up again. This raising and lowering is one repetition. It seems too easy right? Well, truth is that it is in theory, but in practice, to actually recruit the right muscles is harder. So, you will know you have done it correctly once you start to feel the lower abdomen and stomach working.

Repeat this 10 times for 3 sets. If you feel any pain in the neck or in the legs, stop. Don't do any exercise if you feel it is making anything worse.

VIDEO LINK: https://youtu.be/DtbET9HL33g

2. **Side Plank** - the second exercise in the McGill series is harder than you would expect but still has steps and modifications along the way that you can take to make it easier or harder as you get stronger in the core and spine. It is designed to strengthen the muscles on the side of the core called the obliques, these are diagonal shaped muscles that run into the pelvis and low back. When we side bend or twist, these will prevent anything from becoming unstable from the side position (McGill, 2015).

A lot of the time our clients will describe having a problem of bending down to pick something up off the floor, and then when getting back up they felt the back go. This can often be due to weak obliques. They are often not strong enough and don't provide enough support. This is a key muscle to get working optimally.

To start this, lie on your side, your hips level with your torso, so not rotating back or forwards. The elbow is on the ground and propped up at 90 degrees, so you are putting your weight through the elbow. If you have started on your left side, then your left hip will be touching the floor. You want to very slowly contract the left side and feel the muscles tighten from your armpit all the way down to your hip.

Bringing the hip off the floor, you will feel pressure on your shoulder and on the left side of the torso, this is good, you shouldn't feel tension in the back. Then slowly lower the hip back down. At this point, the legs haven't moved, they will be bent at 45 degrees and the hip does all the work.

Repeat this 10 times, 3 sets. This may be too easy, and you aren't feeling it in the side muscles, as you are not putting enough weight through them. So, the next step is to straighten the legs out, putting one foot in front of the other. And then initiate the contraction again but raising the hip and the knee off the floor so all the weight goes through the feet and the shoulder. These are the only two contact points. This is much harder and will generate more strength quicker in the lateral core.

Some teething issues will be pain in the shoulder. Make sure the shoulder is in line with the rest of the body, not too far forwards or rotated backwards.

Another issue is pain in the knee. Again, this can be a torsion issue, so ensure that you aren't rolling forwards, or get someone to watch and make sure there is a straight line from the head to the feet.

With the harder version, you may want to reduce the repetitions that you are doing, so start with 5 and build up to 10 again once feeling comfortable.

VIDEO LINK: https://youtu.be/-cPZejJvaYg

3. **Bird Dog** - this is the third exercise in the McGill series and is the hardest (always leave the hardest to last). This exercise increases stability in the low back. A lot of the time we hear clients say "I just bent down and my back went" or "I just leant to open the window and I dropped to the floor." This is because of a build-up in instability, whether it's in the low back or the pelvis. The ligaments and muscles have a lack of control and cannot support the spine. Over time, they will gradually lose more stability, and as the disc or spinal column will take more load, the body can compensate for this change in load. Until it says enough is enough and can't take the stress on the disc or a delicate structure in the back and will lock everything down to protect it. This could be a spasm and build up of inflammation, and it means you can't move effectively, but it protects the integral structures (McGill, 2015).

What this exercise does is ensure that doesn't happen, it activates and stabilises the ligaments and muscles in the spine. This ensures that the discs and spinal column don't take up extra weight and limits the chance of a spasm occurring.

People with knee pain may struggle with this, as you need to start on all fours. Try it in bed to start with, if that doesn't work, then see the exercise below; it's similar but on the back. It doesn't offer as much stability control but is a great exercise for increasing strength of the core and natural brace.

The beginning of the bird dog is vital. You need to start on all fours with the shoulders over the wrists. Get comfortable and find the 'neutral spine'. What on earth is the neutral spine?

You will tip the hips back and forwards similar to the happy cat exercise above but keep the ribs still. Once you have gone back and forwards several times, then find the 'middle' of those two positions, pull the tummy in and squeeze the bum.

a. First progression is just using the arms, so keeping the torso and hips completely still, just lengthen one arm out in front and come back, then lengthen the other arm and repeat 5 times on each side. All the time keeping the contraction of the tummy and bum muscles and not letting the hips rock from side to side when lifting the arm forwards.

b. Second progression is just using the legs, a little harder as these are heavier. Keeping the tummy tight, squeeze the buttock muscles and lift and extend one leg back, hold it and then do the other one.

c. Third Progression is using both the arms and legs. Don't move to this stage until you feel comfortable with a and b. You need to ensure you are not rocking from side to side and you have one long spine that isn't twisted or moving around. At the same time, lift the left leg and the right arm and extend them both, then return to the original resting position and repeat with the right leg and left arm, so you are working opposites. This increases the tension across the body, so you essentially have two slings that are pulling the body into a good position and supporting your spine.

The 'slings' are vital because when you bend and twist, they will provide enormous support and prevent stress in the spine.

Repeat on each side 5 times, really slowly. Each repetition should take at least 5 seconds. Do 3 sets total.

VIDEO LINK:
https://www.youtube.com/watch?v=jmVMUVbYqQI

4. **Dead bug** - the dead bug is a great exercise to increase the contraction of the 'natural brace' that forms from your stomach all the way round the sides to the back. If you do wear an artificial brace when lifting or

bending, then this will switch off those muscles if it becomes relied upon. They are vital to finding the cure to back pain.

This is also a good alternative to the bird dog if you suffer with knee pain, as there is no weight that goes through the knee as you begin by lying on your back.

You want to start lying on your back with your knees bent at 45 degrees and keep the hands by your side to start with. Similar to the bird dog, you want to start by rocking your hip backwards and forwards and finding the middle ground, and just be aware of where your hips and pelvis are.

Then you will place your hands under your spine and feel a curve or gap there, you want to close this gap up to increase the contraction of the core and pelvic floor. This is done by pulling the tummy button towards the spine and pushing the back down (tough right?).

Then lift the legs up off the floor to 90 degrees and 90 degrees at the knees so you are forming a tabletop, keeping that back flat on the floor. Slowly, let one leg go down towards the floor as you extend it. At the end of the extension, when the leg is getting straight, the low back will want to arch, you have to prevent this from happening, so really squeeze the back and tummy to stop it coming away, then bring the leg back to tabletop position. Repeat with the other side.

This needs to be done very slowly, 5 seconds down, 5 seconds up. If you can only manage one on each side, that is better than doing five quick and not effective repetitions.

The second stage, which I wouldn't recommend until you are happy with the first part, We need to build in the arms. You begin in the same starting position, take the legs up, the right leg will go down as the left arm goes back, then bring them back to the middle and repeat on the other side, all the time keeping that tummy contracted and pulled in.

Repeat another 2 times aiming for 5 repetitions on each side. The key is to keep it as slow as possible.

VIDEO LINK:
https://www.youtube.com/watch?v=uuT7JoiVhF0&t=9s

Corrective Blocks to shape the spine

There is a technique called chiropractic biophysics, which is the most researched technique in chiropractic to date. It was founded by Dr Deed Harrison, and it looks at the shape of the curves in the spine and compares them to normal. What they then do is perform a series of adjustments and use corrective wedges to get the spine as close to its 'normal' position as possible. The results they get are outstanding as shown on a pre and post x-ray. We use corrective wedges in the clinic, think of them like an orthotic in your shoe.

You may have come across orthotics when you were younger or use them now. They support the arches in the feet to give us good stability going forwards with our walking. The spinal corrective wedges act in a similar way. Our clients lie on them in the clinic and at home, and they help to lengthen and restore the normal curves in the spine.

When we look at someone from the front, they need to be straight and the spine should be straight. If we look at someone from the side, then they need to have three curves in the spine for shock absorption and mobility. The neck and low back curve are the same direction and then the thoracic or mid spine is the other way. The most common curve to distort is the neck curve because we sit and use computers or smartphones for too long.

They aren't the most comfortable things in the world, they are designed to be firm so they can change the curves in the spine, no one said this game was easy, I'm sorry. There are various brands and alternatives out there, but Denneroll is the certified orthotic pillow used by CBP and is the most effective. You have to lie on these for at least fifteen minutes in the evening for a period of three months, so if you are going to invest the time, it's worth investing in the best wedge.

With the wedges they need to be used on a hard surface; the bed or sofa does not give enough feedback. Start with 5 minutes and increase it each day by one minute, if it feels comfortable, until you get to 20 minutes. If at any point you feel pain, just stop and get up slowly and let me know info@westchiropractic.co.uk. We can modify it for you to make it suitable.

1. **Lumbar wedge** - so often the lumbar curve can increase, and we call this a hyper-lordosis. Often, people who have this will notice they stick their bums out a lot more, and pregnant women often develop a hyper-lordosis.

    It's a problem, as over time when the curve is increased the rib cage moves backwards and puts more pressure on the spine thus causing pain. You want to lie on the wedge on your buttocks or where you feel the SIT bones (ischial tuberosities). Lift the knees to 45 degrees and lie down on a hard surface, not the mattress or sofa as it doesn't give enough feedback.

    The other way the spine can go in the low back is to become straight and hypo-lordotic. This is problematic for the discs, as they don't have any shock absorption help from the spine and all the weight of the torso and head is going through a 'stiff rod' rather than a bendy spine. This means the discs will take up more load thus causing more pressure on them and making them susceptible to herniation (medical term for a 'slipped disc'.

    So the wedge should go in the small of the back and you should lie back on it. This will feel uncomfortable, and if it is too much, then just bend the knees slightly to ease the pressure on the spine. Once you feel more comfortable after several weeks, you can try and straighten the legs again to get more of a curve back in the spine.

To get up off the lumbar wedge, always roll off to the side and slowly lift yourself up with your hands.

2. **Denneroll/Cervical Wedge -** this is the more commonly applied wedge, as this is the curve that our clients will usually have lost before anything else goes. The reason is due to desk work, smartphones and iPads all putting pressure on the neck and causing people to lean forward. The head is heavy, between 12-15lbs, and the neck is movable so it can't take the strain.

The Denneroll is a smaller and firmer wedge and it is used to regain the curve in the spine when the head hasn't gone as far forward, so if someone has a straight neck, we would usually use this. Same concept as above, start at 5 minutes and build it up.

Often there is some confusion about where to put the Denneroll. Always ask a practitioner, as where you put it will determine the quality of the results. Depending on an x-ray, it may be more beneficial to have the Denneroll further up the neck or closer to the shoulders.

It may cause some discomfort to start with. If it causes a dull headache, just let us know.

The second device is the neck wedge. This is used for clients whose head goes too far forward (anterior head carriage). It is a much bigger wedge and will generate more of an angle as the head falls back off the edge. Again, when coming off this, take care and be slow as you roll off to the side rather than lifting the head up and off.

If you would like further information about our corrective wedges, then please call 01932 355529 and we can arrange a fitting.

The secret remedy to getting rid of back pain for good

The Secret Chalice, Lost Ark & The Mythical Beast.

Resolving back pain, as you have probably gathered by now, is an incredibly difficult challenge for a lot of experts to begin to master. It requires help from an specialist, focus from a patient, and determination to keep persevering even when things are slow.

It is similar to when people sign up to the gym in January with good intentions. They have put on a few pounds and are ready to hit the gym five times a week to get their New Year body shape. What often happens is that even with all the will in the world, it gradually dissipates as the month draws near. There is a lack of progression, no results, and most people will lose interest. Which is why gyms will make up to 70% of their annual revenue in the month of January, due to this new human nature of desiring things instantly, right now, and with one click. We all seem to want everything now and a quick fix.

Very often, when undergoing any sort of back treatment program, whether it be Pilates, physiotherapy, or chiropractic, there tends to be a slow start, particularly with chronic issues that have been going on longer than two years. With more acute issues, for example a disc injury that has happened in the last few days, these will clear up much more quickly, and the patient will experience immediate results. However, it's important to still get to the root cause of the issue as to why it actually happened to prevent it from coming back in the future.

This is the same for both acute and chronic conditions, we have to find out the reason why something is happening to create long-term results. If we constantly chase symptoms and never isolate the root cause of the issue, then it really won't get better, or will get better and then come back in the future.

We had a client come to us called Dave who was a decorator. He had spent the last twenty-five years up on ladders, crouching down, and leaning with his head back painting ceilings. He was suffering with severe migraines for the last four years, which would be so debilitating that he couldn't get out of bed and get to work. The migraine would also come on when he was with his son in the swimming pool, meaning he couldn't spend time with him.

This all got too much when Dave became self-employed, as many tradesmen do, and he was finding that he was having to take too much time off, and it was starting to affect his business. That's when he called us, and we scheduled an initial assessment for him.

When Dave was telling us the story, I naively assumed that he had pressure on the top of his neck, which is where 90% of migraines usually come from. This was going to be an easy case and we would be able to get him back up and running in no time at all.

We began treatment two weeks ago, and he said the migraines were worse than ever, if anything. He was taking more time off work, and he couldn't go on like that. So we sat down and examined him again to analyse why this was happening. I checked his x-rays, and his motion study performed a series muscle tests. We cleared out the issue at the top of his neck where I'd been adjusting more. He was irritating the nerve that was going around his head, causing his headaches to get worse.

Often with headaches and migraines, the pain could come from somewhere else in the body or can be due to another issue. What a lot of our patients find difficult to understand is how integral the jaw is to neck pain and migraines. How can something that is completely irrelevant to the neck and head be the source of their pain?

The jaw has huge amounts of nervous system activity going down it and up to the brain; any deviation or overactivity can have a knock-on effect to the rest of the body. After testing, it was clear as day he was suffering from something called bruxism where he was clenching his teeth while he was sleeping, causing an overactivity of the muscles around the jaw which refers to pain in the head, causing his migraines.

With this, we had to design a mouth guard for him to wear at night so that he would stop the grinding and clenching of his jaw. We adjusted and treated the jaw to set it in the correct position, and within two weeks his headaches had completely disappeared. Dave was back to working full time on his business and spending time with his son.

I would love to say over the next six to nine months of seeing Dave he didn't have one headache again but often with healing in the spine it's just not the case. Dave became complacent and was only wearing his mouth guard three out of seven nights in the week. The jaw became inflamed again. Because of the relationship between the jaw and neck, it's really important to restore the normal function of the neck and shoulders to allow the jaw to operate normally and not become inflamed again. So, as we remodelled his neck, there was obviously still going to be some stress around the jaw which we explained to Dave that it may flare up from time to time but it's still moving in the right direction.

Once the normal neck curve started to come back in Dave's spine, the jaw retracted and set in the joint with no aggravation to the muscles, closing the full resolution of his symptoms. This is so important because if we had kept on treating his neck issue, this problem would have kept coming back and we would never have fully resolved it.

What's the difference between Chiropractors, Osteopaths, and Physiotherapists?

One of the most common questions I receive! When faced with a back or neck issue, many people will often ask this, as in which profession treats each condition better. I have been treated by all three, and you have to remember that the next chapter is biased, as I'm a Chiropractor. But I honestly think all three are great and a cross-referral or multi-disciplinary approach for certain conditions is key.

You often get this in many industries, the 'he said' 'she said' type situation. It doesn't help anybody, and most of all it does not help the patient. We will try and help where we can, but if it's not our condition or we don't manage it as well, then we will always refer out to someone who is better. We have a sports massage therapist in the clinic, and we refer to them a lot, as there are some conditions that we aren't as good with, as them.

For example, if someone comes to see me with a pain in the elbow, we do a full examination and try to find the source of the issue. Often, elbow pain can be referred from the neck and shoulder, so treating the elbow is redundant and won't cause a long term fix, as the problem will keep coming back. We diagnosed a tennis elbow, and although I can help, our sports therapist sees this every day and is much better at treating this, so we refer to him.

As far as the difference, Chiropractic was founded in 1895 in Iowa, Davenport by a man called D.D Palmer. His son B.J Palmer brought Chiropractic to the world and promoted it. Chiropractors work on the basis that the spine is a protective casing for the nervous system. This is the brain and the nerves in the spinal cord going to every single muscle, cell, organ and gland. So, for your heart to beat and lungs to breathe the nervous system has to be working optimally. If it isn't, then the body won't be as healthy as it could be and the person will experience symptoms such as pain, dysfunction, or immobility.

If the spine is ever compromised with stress, for example a fall or accident or sitting in the wrong position for too long, then it can put pressure on the spinal cord and thus the nervous system, affecting its ability to function, and therefore symptoms can appear. We call this a subluxation or misalignment.

This is what Chiropractors are looking to identify and how this affects the spine and the structures around it. Often when we see a subluxation in the low back or pelvis, this will affect how someone is walking and cause more pressure on one knee than the other, thus causing knee pain. If we just treat the knee this is great, but when that person goes back to walking, then the knee pain will come back because of the pressure on the body.

Physiotherapists tend to focus more on the muscles in the body. They use a variety of different techniques to improve the muscle tension and flexibility throughout. They also prescribe detailed exercise rehabilitation programmes to restore mobility and reduce pain. In my experience, they tend to focus on sports injuries like knee and shoulder issues resulting from an injury. They do look at back pain as well, and it just depends on which works best for you. If there is a disc issue resulting from a subluxation, then no amount of muscle work will correct that, as it will keep pulling everything back. It needs to be adjusted first before the muscle work will have a long-term beneficial correction.

Osteopaths sit somewhere in the middle, and they will focus on the circulatory system, to pump more blood around the body. The theory goes that more blood in the body will provide more oxygen and vitamins to certain structures and allow the body to function more closely to optimal. I have been treated by an osteopath and he did very similar adjustments that I would do, although he did admit he had studied a lot of chiropractic and does a lot of adjustments that way. What I have found is that most osteopaths will look at back pain but use a variety of adjustments and muscle work to get results.

The main thing to find out is who best aligns with what you need. Ring the offices and have a chat with the assistant and see what they treat and their specialities. For us it's low back, neck pain, and sciatica. This is what we see every day and love treating, as we get great results for our patients. If someone comes with an ankle issue from a walking injury, we will always have a look for them but then either refer them to our sports massage therapist or out to a physio.

When you ring, you will want to ask what the initial process is. Do they perform a full examination, medical history, and do they take x-rays to find out the root cause of the issue?

I'm too old to get my back fixed

Something we often hear is "I'm too old for chiropractic, I'm too past it and you can't help me." Why do people think this way? Because a lot of the time, the older population have tried a number of things and suffered with pains for ten or twenty, even thirty plus years. They are sceptical, and they are reluctant to try anything else because all the methods before have failed. I completely understand; if I had tried painkillers, hot baths and massage with no resolution of my pain and to be told by a medical doctor that this is something that has to be lived with and managed, then I would be reluctant to try something new as well.

I want to tell you a story about a recent client that came to us called James. James was one of the most incredible 86-year olds I've had the pleasure of meeting. Although I didn't realise that until he finished his corrective care plan with us.

Let me explain, James came to us with his daughter, and he was in severe pain. He had sciatica for the last two months and could barely speak. We couldn't do an examination because he couldn't lie down or sit, and we had to take the case history standing up. We just about got some x-rays taken, and it was clear why he was getting sciatica. He had osteoarthritis at the base of his spine which was causing compression of the bottom nerve which runs down the leg, called the sciatic nerve.

The main thing for James was that he couldn't care for his wife who was suffering with dementia. This meant that the rest of the family had to take shifts to look after James but also James' wife. Remember, back pain doesn't just affect the individual, it also affects the ones close to them as well.

James is incredibly independent, still doing loads of DIY, gardening, and caring for the both of them. However, since the sciatica started, he was sleeping downstairs in the front room on the floor, as it was the only place that was comfortable, unable to look after his wife. As someone who takes incredible pride in how he's presented, he wasn't even getting dressed to start the day (although I must say, when we first met he was wearing a suit and tie, that's dedication).

When we went through the results with James and the family, I told him that we can't correct osteoarthritis, but we can take pressure off the nerve to get rid of the sciatica, but the change in the shape of the bone had been there too long. They were happy about that and let me begin treatment.

It was slow to begin with and James was seeing us twice a week. The reason for twice a week is that we don't allow the spine to go back to the position it wanted to be in so we can keep building on each adjustment, to change the spine long-term and cause resolution.

It wasn't until week three, James came in and pretty much skipped onto the bed. Dr Geoffrey and I couldn't believe it, we thought it would take a lot longer due to his age and the level of damage in the base of his spine. But it goes to show that everyone is different.

It was a complete turn-around for him and the family, and I'm glad to say that he is back home looking after his lovely wife and normality has been restored for James and his family.

On the opposite end of the scale, we often get clients asking us "What is the youngest patient you have?" We have seen babies as young as six months in the clinic. A lot of people seem confused by this and think Chiropractors can only help people with bad backs. We focus on the nervous system and optimise that to ensure everything is working.

With new-borns, they have often had a traumatic birth and their start in life can be harder. For example, forceps delivery can put pressure on the cranial bones. This can affect the neck and jaw and can cause problems with sleeping or ability to latch on whilst feeding.

It's so important to give babies the best start in life. My son, now fourteen months, had a ventouse delivery, which is a suction cup on his head. He had a cone shaped head for the first twenty-four hours before the swelling settled down. What this did though is pull the top part of his neck, and he found it difficult to lie on one side and latch on when feeding on that side. We started doing some cranial work on him and he settled down once the tension started to reduce. He seemed to become much more comfortable.

The Most Common Questions my Clients Ask

What's the best way to pick my kids up?

This is something that I have completely neglected until the last year. We had a baby last year, and I always thought to myself, how can something so small cause so many issues with people's spines? Well I have to say, I was very quickly humbled. Reading stories, feeding and picking him up has taken its toll on my spine. As I mentioned earlier, I suffer with disc issues in my low back, and with sleep deprivation we completely neglect our bodies and forget to look after ourselves. I would find myself picking him up, lifting him up over the cot and straining my low back with the leverage. Also, holding him to be fed was putting pressure on my neck and upper back, being in that position for forty-five minutes or more is a sustained compression through the spine.

Now, at the time of writing this, he is fourteen months, and it's easier as he is more mobile, but we still lift him out of the pram and the cot. The main issue I see is bending down into the cot, as we lean over and stress the low back when picking up. So, my solution to this is to squat and bend the knees before bending over, taking as much leverage in the glutes and legs before picking the child up. Then squeeze the tummy and core and try and bring them as close to you as possible before actually lifting them up. When you initiate the lift, squeeze everything and slowly extend the back whilst squeezing the bum. If they are too far apart and you try to do this, then this is when we can cause too much leverage on the low spine and can cause back issues.

Whilst we are on the kids topic, when feeding, this is mainly for the mums, it's so important to try and keep the shoulder blades back and down and the head up. All too often we see many new mum's come in with neck and shoulder issues caused by feeding.

Should I have surgery?

This should be the absolute last resort. Spinal surgeons will reluctantly do surgery, as they know the risks (Schaller, 2004). Often people stay the same or get worse. I have seen some clients in sheer agony and unable to move for months on end; it is completely destroying their lives. At this stage, often there is little we can do as Chiropractors, or not enough to make it worth carrying on with the pain for another six months. When there is stenosis, which is a narrowing of the spinal canal, or so much instability that it would be unsafe to try and correct through adjustments, then we would refer to a spinal surgeon. Usually, most people will feel an immediate benefit. The issue with spinal surgery is because you get that initial benefit then patients forget they still need to look after their spine with exercises and core stability training. They then end up back in a similar situation years down the line. Pain is our only indicator of how healthy our spine is, and when it goes, we think everything is fine.

Discectomy is a surgery that I'm not keen on, the reason being when someone has disc pain usually it can be solved non-surgically with care and rehabilitation. Some surgeons are keen to do this as it will provide immediate relief but long-term, what is the health of that spine? Where is the rest of the pressure going? What are the future results going to yield?

Why do golfers love chiropractic?

Based in West Byfleet, we do see a number of golfers due to the sheer number of clubs around us. Golf is a great sport, a true test of mental and physical fitness. I'm amazed at the four hours of immense concentration and the mental battle with yourself that golf requires of people, a true test of character. Let alone the professionals playing eighteen holes every day for four days in a tournament with immense pressure.

We see many golfers because of the nature of the sport; there is a lot of twisting in the swing. Mainly the longer shots demand more power to be generated through the torso, thus causing disc strain. You only have to look at Tiger Woods and see the health of his spine. He has been in and out of surgery for the last ten years. Almost ended his career, only to come back and win a Major Championship. Incredible.

The twisting movement doesn't need to cause problems in the back though, you can still generate enough power and torque to drive the ball a long way without causing damage to the discs. This is done by increasing the strength of the midline and also the obliques so that when you twist it goes through the muscles and they protect the spine. The best place to start is the side plank exercise mentioned previously, this is great at generating strength and stability in the side of the body and great for golfers.

Most core exercises will help golfers and reduce back pain. The main aim is to get through eighteen holes pain-free forever, get to the 19th and enjoy your time after, rather than having to pop painkillers or get straight in the car to lie down.

What is a decompression table?

We have many resources available to us in the clinic including a digital x-ray machine, shockwave therapy, massage therapy, plus four Chiropractors. The decompression table is a state-of-the-art machine that is one of the most effective ways of relieving pressure on a disc either in the neck or the low back without using surgery (Choi *et al*, 2015).

Our clients use the decompression table frequently when they are suffering with a disc herniation. It instantly relieves pressure by applying traction to the spinal segments either side of the disc away from each other, reducing pressure and pain in the spine and often sciatic pain.

If you would like to know more about our decompression therapy, then please call us on 01932 355529.

What do our clients say

"West Chiropractic is a fantastic place. From initial assessment through to the treatment and the amazing support staff they have it really is an incredible practise. The information you get is detailed and thorough and the personal approach makes you feel they really are treating you as an individual. I cannot rate them enough they have managed in a very short time to change a long term issue in my back and provided good advice for maintaining it in the future, who knew not having constant back pain could be so life altering! The team are amazing and it's so refreshing to go somewhere where the service in all aspects is 5*."

"I've been visiting this chiropractic clinic for a number of months now after many sleepless nights due to upper and lower back pain. Antonio has set me on the right path to correcting my spine and posture which as a result has diminished all pain that I had. Jeremy runs an amazing clinic here with a great team behind him. Everybody is friendly with a great wealth of knowledge. Would definitely recommend."

"Having recently moved to the area, I was keen to restart Chiropractic care with a local practitioner and having found West Chiropractic have been undergoing a 3 month course to help set a course for future wellbeing. I have found the entire team very friendly and accommodating, making me feel very welcome on each visit.

The original observation session was very revealing and made it all the more apparent the need for chiropractic care. The explanation was made easy to understand and he goal setting by myself was converted into medical goal setting by Jeremy.

Not all facilities have the equipment that West Chiropractic possess so that is an advantage in itself.

I'm looking forward to continuing to see the improvements made so far."

"West Chiropractic are a professional, friendly team who have totally relieved my neck pain with the treatment plan that Jeremy advised.

It is a pleasure to go to an appointment and be greeted by the smiling faces of the admin team.

I now have an ongoing regular maintenance treatment plan and consider this to be the best way of investing in my health and well being."

"I would definitely recommend West Chiropractic if you think you need some adjustments done with your body. All the staff are easy to talk to and I feel very safe any time I am there. It's such a warm and lovely atmosphere too. Oh, and the music playlist is always good too. Worth every penny!"

"My son and I feel truly blessed to have found West Chiropractor. I've never met such a great bunch of friendly and lovely people! So welcoming. We have had a huge improvement and feel so much better. I highly recommend West Chiropractic, you will be in the best hands! Thank you for having my back!"

How To Start Your Recovery TODAY by claiming a completely FREE diagnostic "Discovery Session" with a Chiropractor...

Step one in the recovery from ANY back pain is to actually get to the true, underlying root cause. Without knowing what's going wrong it's almost impossible to stop it long term. Getting to the "true, underlying, root cause of back pain" is something that a Chiropractor works to do... and it's a shame that some people still don't know how easy it is to "self-refer" to a Chiropractor for help with back pain. No Referral From A Doctor is Needed... How easy? Well, there's NO one to ask, NO referral needed, NO forms to sign, NO payment agreements and there's NO obligation to go ahead with any Chiropractic care after an initial consultation which will reveal your "diagnosis" – i.e. the, what's going wrong to cause your pain in the first place!

It's true... you don't even need a referral from a medical doctor. This means you can just call up and arrange that first DISCOVERY VISIT - today if you like, and likely have answers within the next 48 hours! It's that easy. And at that first DISCOVERY CONSULTATION with one of my Chiropractors, you can have all of your questions answered personally, one who WILL also find out what's going wrong and what else can be done about it, and by who... to get you there faster! Then, once you know that, you're better able to decide whether or not to go ahead or what to do.

What I'm offering you is called a DISCOVERY VISIT... because you get to discover all about YOU, YOUR BACK

PAIN, "US" (the friendly staff at West Chiropractic!), AND Chiropractic. You'd leave your FREE Discovery Session knowing what's causing your back pain and able to make a better, more educated and more informed decision about your health! Offering this is why I say Chiropractic could be a "hassle free" way of easing knee pain - it's financially risk free because the first visit is 100% FREE.

Published by Dr Jeremy Andrews (Doctor of Chiropractic). Here's how you make contact with us and take advantage of this FREE Discovery Visit: To talk to Jeremy about your back pain, Just call: 01932 355529 or Email: info@westchiropractic.co.uk

And At That First Discovery Session, Here's What You Will "Discover":

1. What is the underlying root cause of your pain and the real reason your suffering?
2. Can Chiropractic help YOU?
3. If YES, exactly what sort of recovery program do you need?
4. How long before you will experience positive results?
5. Are there any OTHER natural healing, drug free ways you can exploit to speed up your recovery alongside Chiropractic?
6. What your recovery program will likely cost.
7. How soon you can do gentle exercise, get back to work, or enjoy play time again with your family and even walk with friends or stand in line at the shops.

References

A study of work stress, patient handling activities and the risk of low back pain among nurses in Hong Kong- Yin bing Yip, 2001

Failed back surgery syndrome: the role of symptomatic segmental single-level instability after lumbar microdiscectomy- B. Schaller, 2004

Influences of spinal decompression therapy and general traction therapy on the pain, disability, and straight leg raising of patients with intervertebral disc herniation- Jioun Choi, Sangyong Lee, Gak Hwangbo, 2015

Low back disorders: evidence-based prevention and rehabilitation- Stuart McGill, 2015

Reduction of progressive thoracolumbar adolescent idiopathic scoliosis by chiropractic biophysics® (CBP®) mirror image® methods following failed traditional chiropractic treatment: a case report- Joshua S. Haggard, Jennifer B. Haggard, Paul A. Oakley and Deed E. Harrison- 2017

What We Can Learn About Running from Barefoot Running: An Evolutionary Medical Perspective- Lieberman, Daniel E, 2012

Yoga and Pilates in the management of low back pain- Susan Sorosky, Sonja Stilp & Venu Akuthota, 2007

Printed in Great Britain
by Amazon